Atlas of Normal Roentgen Variants That May Simulate Disease

Other Books by Theodore E. Keats

An Atlas of Normal Developmental Roentgen Anatomy,
Second Edition, with Thomas A. Smith

Emergency Radiology

Atlas of Roentgenographic Measurement,
Sixth Edition

Radiology of Musculoskeletal Stress Injury

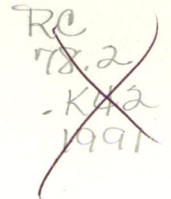
FIFTH EDITION

Atlas of Normal Roentgen Variants That May Simulate Disease

THEODORE E. KEATS, M.D.
Professor and Chairman
Department of Radiology
University of Virginia School of Medicine
Charlottesville, Virginia

Mosby
Year Book

St. Louis   Baltimore   Boston   Chicago   London   Philadelphia   Sydney   Toronto

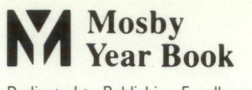 Mosby
Year Book

Dedicated to Publishing Excellence

Sponsoring Editor: Anne S. Patterson
Assistant Editor: Dana Battaglia
Associate Managing Editor, Manuscript Services: Deborah Thorp
Production Coordinator: Nancy C. Baker
Proofroom Manager: Barbara Kelly

1 2 3 4 5 6 7 8 9 0 CL/AK 96 95 94 93 92

Library of Congress Cataloging-in-Publication Data
Keats, Theodore E. (Theodore Eliot), 1924-
    Atlas of normal roentgen variants that may simulate disease /
Theodore E. Keats.—5th ed.
      p.   cm.
    Includes bibliographical references and index.
    ISBN 0-8151-5048-2
    1. Radiography, Medical—Atlases. 2. Diagnostic errors—Atlases.
I. Title.
    [DNLM: 1. Radiography—atlases. WN 17 K25a]
RC78.2.K42 1991
616.07′572—dc20   91-21936
DNLM/DLC   CIP
for Library of Congress

To Dr. John F. Holt—Teacher, friend, and the source of inspiration for this work

Foreword

My interest in anatomic variants dates back to World War II when, as a young 4-F Instructor in Radiology, it was my duty to intercept residents' film-reading queries on the way to "The Chief," hoping to save precious moments for our one and only professor, who was swamped with countless administrative problems in those days of severe manpower shortage. Eventually I kept score and discovered that, during one three-month period, the questions brought up by residents and fellow staff members regarding anatomic and physiologic variants outnumbered those concerning pathologic entities by three to one. Admittedly, a few of the aberrations that we initially thought to be variants eventually proved to be pathologic in nature, but the converse was true far more often, so I am reasonably certain that this ratio is at least as high today as it was thirty years ago.

When Caffey's classic text, *Pediatric X-Ray Diagnosis,* appeared in 1945 with its novel emphasis on anatomic variations, my interest in the subject was spurred again. In ensuing conversations and correspondence, Dr. Caffey repeatedly emphasized the great need for a comprehensive text on variants and artifacts encompassing both children and adults. He urged me to undertake the project alone, while generously offering his own collection of pediatric variants for my use in any way I saw fit. Subsequent informal discussions, lectures, and instruction courses at national meetings on my part clearly supported Caffey's convictions. Preliminary plans for the book were formulated and the gathering of additional material was begun.

Despite encouragement and support from all sides, this project did not reach fruition. There are a number of reasons why this was so, but one in particular stands out. As the collection of variants progressed in the form of films, negatives, photographic prints, and countless notations in books and on cards, it became first a steamroller and then an avalanche, resulting in eventual disorganization and utter frustration. No cutoff point ever came clearly into view, and the book became unaffectionately known as "The Monster." It was with a feeling of great relief that I happily relinquished any claims I had on the book to the eager and able hands of Ted Keats, former resident and longtime close friend, who had been quietly assembling his own collection of variants over the years.

Keats has neatly and effectively sidestepped my dilemma in several ways. Rather than trying to present all possible variants of the paranasal sinuses, the sella turcica, or the small intestine (just to cite three of many possible examples), he has wisely included only those which truly simulate recognizable disease entities. In so doing he has avoided the impossible and, more important, has brought the subject into practical perspective and has spared the reader much irrelevant trivia. His use of the atlas format in dealing with this material is also to be commended. The old argument that an atlas automatically precludes true scholarly achievement is just not valid in many aspects of diagnostic roentgenology and is nicely refuted by this particular volume. The carefully selected roentgenograms that have been so meticulously reproduced herein speak for themselves in a most eloquent manner.

Congratulations, Ted, on a job well done.

JOHN F. HOLT, M.D.
Co-Director, Division of Pediatric Radiology (Retired)
C. S. Mott Children's Hospital
University of Michigan Medical Center
Ann Arbor, Michigan

Preface to the Fifth Edition

Say not "This is the truth" but "So it seems to me to be as I now see the things I think I see."

Inscription above a doorway at the German Naval Officers School in Kiel, quoted by John McPhee in *Rising From the Plains*

The many expressions of acceptance of this work have been most gratifying and have provided me with the stimulus to continue to collect and explain many of the normal phenomena that we see in our everyday work.

As I have collected normal roentgen variants over the years, I have heard the repeated criticism that the material is unproven, and in many cases the comment is true. Exploration of findings that are unrelated to symptomatology is not a usual undertaking. The quote above states the situation exactly. The inclusion of what I present is often based largely on the fact that the findings are incidental and asymptomatic, or have been seen repeatedly in other patients in a similar clinical setting. In the first edition, I stated that all entries are subject to further scrutiny and exclusion if necessary. I am delighted to state that over the years only a few have failed to survive the test of time.

In this edition I have included more CT images and some MR examinations to establish the developmental nature of some of the new entries. Unfortunately, not many incidental findings are subjected to these kinds of examinations, and only time will permit further documentation.

Mother Nature is inexhaustible in the infinite variety of human development she provides. Since this edition has gone to press, I have collected a great number of new variants for subsequent publications. The task is endless, but it is a labor of love.

I would like to express my appreciation to the many physicians who have sent me material and have graciously granted permission to publish these images. I would like to particularly acowledge the invaluable expertise of Dr. Evan A. Lennon of Sydney, Australia, for his careful proofreading of the manuscript. Thanks are also due to my secretary, Patricia West; my editorial assistant, Carol Chowdhry, Ph.D.; and my wife, Patt, for her encouragement in this work.

THEODORE E. KEATS, M.D.

Preface to the Fourth Edition

To study the phenomena of disease without books is to sail an unchartered sea, while to study books without patients is not to go to sea at all.

Sir William Osler

The publication of this fourth edition reflects the gratifying response of the medical profession to the earlier editions. I have been particularly rewarded by the comments of many radiologists who have indicated that the illustration of these many normal variants has been of great help in their clinical work and in convincing their clinical colleagues of the innocent nature of these findings. I have compiled most of the new entries during the course of my day's work when I can examine and question patients and try to document the nature of the radiographic findings.

Most of the entities in the last edition have stood the test of time. I have removed the illustration of what I believed to be the nutrient foramen of the tibia since I became aware of the typical appearance of the posterior tibial runners' stress fracture. This illustration has been replaced with a correct version. I have added a great deal of new material on the cervical spine. I find this portion of the skeleton extremely difficult to interpret and full of pitfalls for the unwary radiologist, not only because of its anatomic structure, but also as a result of faulty positioning and projection.

The reader will also find some important new material concerning relationships of joints, particularly in the wrist and the acromioclavicular joint, that violate accepted criteria.

I wish to express my appreciation to the many physicians who have permitted me to publish material sent for consultation. I wish to express special appreciation to Dr. Christian Cimmino, of Fredericksburg, Virginia, for his many contributions and his invaluable assistance in unraveling many anatomic riddles. Thanks are also due my secretary, Patricia West; my editorial assistant, Carol Chowdhry; and my wife, Patt, for making my task easier.

THEODORE E. KEATS, M.D.

Preface to the First Edition

The problem of normal variation is a lifelong one for the radiologist, and the mark of his experience is often his ability to recognize a wide range of these entities. Cataloging and describing normal variants demonstrated by roentgenology is of more than academic interest, for recognition of the abnormal first requires full knowledge of the normal. Variation is inseparably related to the study of normal anatomy. In addition, the error of overdiagnosis of a normal variation as evidence of pathology may be more serious than omission and may lead to needless and harmful therapy.

When one studies the field of normal variation in detail, he is apt to be overwhelmed by the seemingly infinite variety nature has provided. A detailed study of all of these would be a valuable, but limitless, undertaking. Of more significance are those variations that may simulate disease in the radiograph. It is these variations that form the substance of this initial effort. Those that are shown here represent problems in diagnosis based on my personal experience, on that of my associates as well as on that of successive generations of residents in training. An interest in the subject of normal variations seems to induce spontaneous generation of additional entities so that, at the time of this writing, there appears to be no end in sight, but it is necessary to make a start. It is anticipated that subsequent editions will add additional troublesome variants as well as correct or amplify those herein as new information is obtained.

The distinction between a normal anatomic variation and a congenital anomaly is an arbitrary one. I have tried to avoid inclusion of anomalies of development, which are obvious in themselves and often productive of signs and symptoms, but rather have tried to concentrate on those alterations that are essentially incidental findings and significant only in their potential for misinterpretation.

The proof of the validity of the material presented is largely subjective, based on personal experience and on the published work of others. It consists largely of having seen the entity many times and of being secure in the knowledge that time has proved the innocence of the lesions. In other cases, follow-up studies indicated that the lesion in question represents a phase of growth that is eliminated by maturation. Still other variants were detected in examination of the side opposite that in question when a radiograph was made for purposes of comparison. Further experience may prove some of these concepts incorrect; all are, therefore, considered subject to future modification or elimination.

This book is arranged in atlas form with the concept that a photographic reproduction of a normal variant is far superior to a text description. The illustrative material, therefore, is emphasized and the text minimal and concise. References are included where the subject is still considered controversial or where documentation is thought necessary. The interested reader is referred to the works *Pediatric X-Ray Diagnosis* by John Caffey and Dr. Alban Kohler's *Borderlands of the Normal and Early Pathologic in Skeletal Roentgenology*. These books represent pioneer efforts in the field of skeletal roentgen variants. This atlas confines itself to roentgen variants seen in conventional roentgenology with no attempt to include those encountered in the specialized fields of angiocardiography, neuroradiology, or the other radiologic specialties. The latter will provide a fruitful source for future study.

Included are a number of normal entities that simulate pathology by virtue of growth, or projection, or both. These are not anatomic variations in the true sense, but since they introduce a similar problem, they are included as well.

The atlas is arranged by anatomic areas. However, certain specific entities are repeated in more than one section, so the reader searching for a variant may encounter it not only in the anatomic area of its origin, but also in the anatomic section of the lesion it simulates. It is hoped this repetitive arrangement will facilitate recognition, particularly for the less experienced observer.

Special acknowledgement is due to Dr. John F. Holt, Professor of Radiology at the University of Michigan, who, as my teacher, first interested me in the subject of normal variation. Throughout his professional career, he has been a student of the subject and has graciously contributed his collection of variants for inclusion in this work. He has also generously contributed time and constructive criticism during the development of this atlas. Without his inspiration and help this work could not have been accomplished.

I wish to express my appreciation also to the many unnamed physicians who have contributed to this collection and, in particular, to Drs. Christian Cimmino and Donald Kenneweg of Fredericksburg, Virginia, and Drs. William R. Newman and Clinton L. Rogers of Cumberland, Maryland, for many valuable cases. My thanks, too, to Miss Anne Russell, R.B.P., of the Section of Medical Photography at the University of Virginia, for her invaluable help in the preparation of the illustrations and to my secretary, Miss Ann Rutledge, for her patience and aid in manuscript preparation.

THEODORE E. KEATS, M.D.

Contents

The Bones

Chapter 1

The Skull

FIG 1–1.— The relative proportions of the cranial vault size to face size in the infant differ strikingly from those of the adult and may suggest a disproportionate increase in vault size in the infant if adult standards are applied. At birth the head-to-face ratio is approximately 4:1. In adults this ratio is 3:2. (Ref: Watson EH, Lowrey GH: *Growth and Development of Children*, ed 5. St Louis, Mosby–Year Book, 1967.) (From Keats TE: Pediatric radiology: Some potentially misleading variations from the adult. *VA Med* 1966; 96:630. Used by permission.)

FIG 1–2.—Overlapping sutures in a neonate secondary to molding of labor.

FIG 1–3.—Scalp folds in a neonate, producing an unusual appearance in the parietal region.

FIG 1–4.—Occipital skin folds.

FIG 1–6.—Hair braids producing an unusual shadow at vertex of skull.

FIG 1–7.—Striations over the parietal area due to hair.

FIG 1–8.—Hair braids with surrounding elastic bands, simulating sclerotic lesions.

FIG 1–9.—Multiple small hair braids ("corn rows"), producing unusual shadows in the frontal and parietal areas.

FIG 1–10.—Hair arrangements—in these two cases a ponytail—may produce unusual shadows.

FIG 1–11.—Two examples of prominent but normal diploic pattern of the calvarium.

FIG 1–12.—Localized prominent diploic pattern in the parietal bone (**A**) produces a striking appearance in Waters projection (**B**).

FIG 1–13.—Irregularities and striations in the vertex of the parietal bone due to the serrations of the sagittal suture. **A,** neonate; **B,** 19-year-old man. (Ref: Sawar M, et al: Nature of vertex striations on lateral skull radiographs. *Radiology* 1983; 146:90.)

FIG 1–14.—Prominent digital markings. The prominence of calvarial digital markings varies widely, particularly between the fourth and tenth years. They do not, in themselves, necessarily reflect increased intracranial pressure. (Ref: Macaulay D: Digital markings in the radiographs of children. *Br J Radiol* 1951; 24:637). It should be noted that infants may occasionally be born without neurologic disease, but having lacunar skull, which will resolve spontaneously. (Ref: Taylor B, Barnat HB, Seibert JJ: Neonatal lacunar skull without neurologic disease. *South Med J* 1982; 75:875.)

FIG 1–15.—Vascular channels in the parietal bone, simulating button sequestra.

FIG 1–17.— Prominent diploic vascular pattern in a child.

FIG 1–18.— Unusual calvarial vascular pattern, simulating fractures.

FIG 1–19.— Two examples of multiple diploic venous lakes, which may simulate metastatic neoplasm. Both patients showed no change on long-term follow-up.

FIG 1–20.—Two examples of prominent, but normal, diploic vascular patterns.

FIG 1–21.—A prominent, but normal, groove for the sphenoparietal venous sinus.

FIG 1–22.—Prominent venous vascular groove at vertex of skull.

FIG 1–23.—Vascular groove (sphenoparietal sinus), simulating fracture.

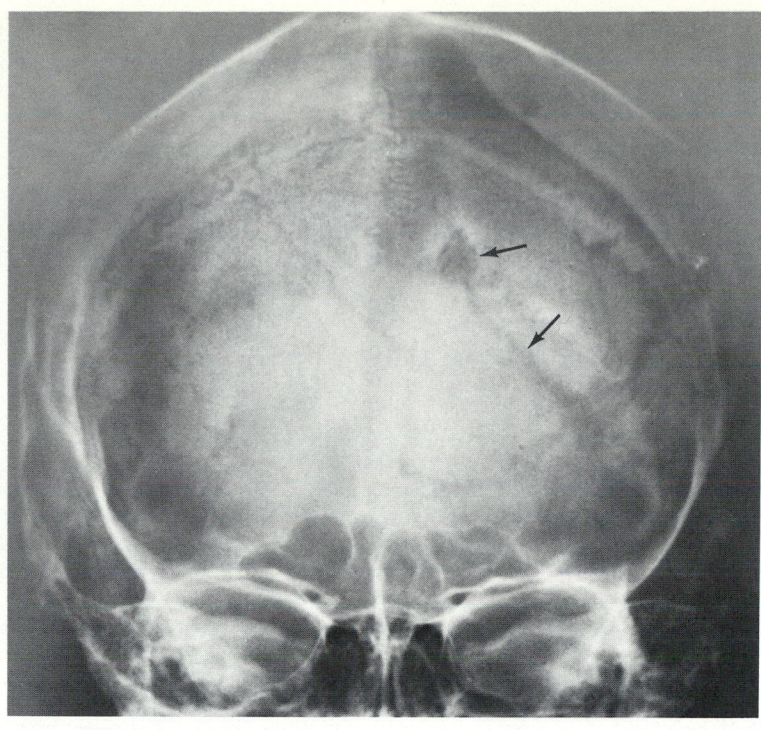

FIG 1–24.—Venous vascular groove in the frontal bone, which may be mistaken for fracture.

FIG 1–25.—Lucent depression of a pacchionian granulation with a large draining vein.

FIG 1–26.—A rather poorly defined pacchionian depression, simulating a destructive lesion, particularly in the lateral projection. (Ref: Branan R, Wilson CB: Arachnoid granulations simulating osteolytic lesions of the calvarium. *AJR* 1976; 127:523.)

FIG 1–27.—Deep, but typical, pacchionian depressions. The external table of the calvarium is bowed, and the internal table is apparently absent. Failure to appreciate these features may lead to an erroneous diagnosis of erosion of the inner table of the skull.

FIG 1–28.—Typical pacchionian depression in the frontal bone. In the frontal view this lucency is often mistaken for a destructive lesion.

FIG 1–29.—Pacchionian depressions in the occipital bone, an unusual location for this normal entity.

FIG 1–30.—Pacchionian depression with a central area of density. This appearance is often mistaken for a significant lesion such as an eosinophilic granuloma. (Ref: Branan R, Wilson CB: Arachnoid granulations simulating osteolytic lesions of the calvarium. *AJR* 1976; 127:523.)

FIG 1–31.—Large pacchionian granulations of the vertex of the skull, lending an unusual configuration to the vertex.

FIG 1–32.—Anterior fontanel bone.

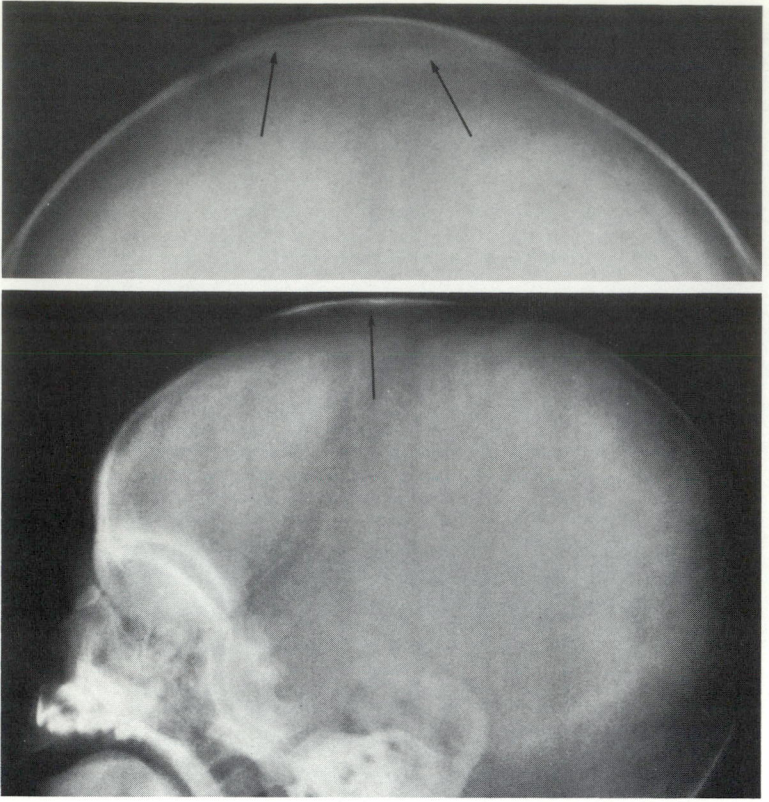

FIG 1–33.—Huge anterior fontanel bone in a 1-month-old child.

FIG 1–34.—Fusing anterior fontanel bone in a 3-year-old boy. This appearance may be confused with a depressed fracture in the lateral projection. (Ref: Girdany BR, Blank E: Anterior fontanel bones. *AJR* 1965; 95:148.)

FIG 1–35.—Anterior fontanel bone in a 5-year-old boy. Note its characteristic appearance in Towne projection.

FIG 1–36.—Closing anterior fontanel bone in an 11-year-old boy.

FIG 1–37.—Remnants of the anterior fontanel bone in a 50-year-old man.

FIG 1–38.—Wormian (sutural) bones in a 7-year-old child. These may be seen as a normal variant as well as in osteogenesis imperfecta and cleidocranial dysostosis.

FIG 1–39.—Wormian bones in a 9-year-old boy.

FIG 1–40.— Wormian bones in a 19-year-old man.

FIG 1–41.— The zygomaticofrontal suture in a neo-nate.

FIG 1–42.— Wormian bones at base of the coronal suture in a newborn (epi-teric bones).

FIG 1–43.— Simulated spread of the coronal sutures in a 4-year-old boy. Sutural prominence is extremely variable, particularly from ages 4 to 8, and should not be mistaken for evidence of increased intracranial pressure. Such early perisutural sclerosis accentuates the prominence of the sutures.

FIG 1–44.—Simulated spread sutures in an 8-year-old boy.

FIG 1–45.—Normal squamosal suture projected tangentially, simulating a fracture.

FIG 1–46.—Tangential projection of squamosal suture, producing less obvious simulated fracture.

FIG 1–47.—The posterior portion of the squamosal suture, which may simulate a fracture, particularly in the lateral projection.

FIG 1–48.—Normal sutural sclerosis of the squamosal suture.

FIG 1–49.—Normal sutural sclerosis of the coronal suture.

FIG 1–50.—Early sutural sclerosis in a 12-year-old boy.

FIG 1–51.—Thick, but normal, calvarium in a 30-year-old man.

FIG 1–52.—Normal frontal, temporal, and occipital lucencies seen in the aging calvarium.

FIG 1–53.—Striking occipital radiolucency in a 32-year-old woman. These localized normal radiolucencies should not be mistaken for osteoporosis circumscripta of Paget's disease.

FIG 1–54.—Generalized and frontal benign cranial hyperostosis in a 38-year-old woman.

FIG 1–55.—Benign cranial hyperostosis in a 65-year-old woman. Diffuse thickening of the calvarium is present as well as localized internal hyperostosis of the frontal and parietal bones.

FIG 1–56.—Frontal and temporal benign cranial hyperostosis in an 81-year-old woman.

FIG 1–57.—*Top left* and *right,* diffuse intracranial hyperostosis in an 88-year-old woman. The radiolucencies were misinterpreted as metastatic deposits. *Bottom right,* CT section shows the radiolucencies due to intervening areas between the hyperostoses.

FIG 1–58.—Localized thickening of the occiptal bone, a normal variation.

FIG 1–59.—Localized thickening of the parietal bone, a normal variation.

FIG 1–60.—Cranium bifidum occultum. Incomplete closure of the midline of the skull in a 7-year-old boy, not to be mistaken for a destructive process. Such closure defects may be unassociated with bone dysplasia. (See Figs 1–95 to 1–99.) (Ref. Inoue Y, et al: Cranium bifidum occultum. *Neuroradiology* 1983; 25:217.)

FIG 1–61.—Localized palpable thinning of the outer table of the skull in an asymptomatic 21-year-old woman. This probably represents an incomplete form of cranium bifidum occultum (see Fig 1–60).

FIG 1–62.—Congenital depressions of the calvarium due to faulty fetal packing. Such depressions present at birth and not associated with edema or hemorrhage of the overlying soft tissues are usually due to faulty position with long-standing pressure from the fetal feet or maternal sacral promontory. (Ref: Caffey J: *Pediatric X-Ray Diagnosis,* ed 8. St Louis, Mosby–Year Book, 1985, p 63; and Eisenberg D, Kirchner SG, Perrin EC: Neonatal skull depressions unassociated with birth trauma. *AJR* 1984; 143:1063.)

FIG 1–63.—Slight calvarial depressions in an 18-month-old-child, probably representing residuals of faulty fetal packing. These depressions usually regress spontaneously without treatment.

FIG 1–64.—Three examples of "doughnut lesions." These are not clinically significant and may be seen in any part of the calvarium, including juvenile skulls. They may or may not contain a central area of sclerosis. (Ref: Keats TE, Holt JF: The calvarial "doughnut lesion": A previously undescribed entity. *AJR* 1969; 105:314.)

FIG 1–65.—The habenular commissure (←) and the pineal gland (←).

FIG 1–66.—Large cystic pineal gland in a 60-year-old man. This finding in itself is of no clinical significance.

FIG 1–67.—Petroclinoid ligament with heavy calcification.

FIG 1–68.— Petroclinoid calcification in the half-axial projection.

FIG 1–69.—Petroclinoid ligament with irregular calcification.

FIG 1–70.—Petroclinoid ligament with unusual pattern of calcification.

FIG 1–71.—Two examples of calcification between the middle and posterior clinoid processes.

FIG 1–72.—Unusual dural calcifications above anterior and posterior clinoid processes.

FIG 1–73.—The os supra petrosum of Meckel, a physiologic calcification under, or adherent to, the dura on the anteroposterior surface of the petrous bone, near its tip. Note its position in the lateral projection, superimposed on the sella turcica, which permits its differentiation from petroclinoid ligament calcification. (Refs: Currarino G, Weinberg A: Os supra petrosum of Meckel. *AJR* 1974; 121:139; and Keats TE: The os supra petrosum of Meckel and nodular petroclinoid ligament calcification. *Va Med* 1977; 104:114.)

FIG 1–74.—The os supra petrosum of Meckel, seen by polytomography.

FIG 1–75.—Prominent frontal crest on the internal surface of the frontal bone, simulating calcification of the falx cerebri in a healthy 4-year-old boy.

FIG 1–76.—Localized focal dural calcification in the parietal area.

FIG 1–77.—Localized focal dural calcification in the frontal area.

FIG 1–78.—Multiple focal areas of dural calcification in a 71-year-old man.

FIG 1–79.—Small localized focal dural calcification in the frontal area.

FIG 1–80.—Calcification of the falx cerebri.

FIG 1–81.—Heavy calcification of the falx cerebri.

FIG 1-82.—Heavy calcification in the falx in frontal and lateral projections.

FIG 1-83.—Three types of physiologic calcification. Demonstrated are petroclinoid ligament (←), heavy calcification of the tentorium cerebelli (⊬), and falx cerebri (⧧).

FIG 1-84.—Minor calcification of the tentorium cerebelli (←). Calcification is also present in the falx (⊬) and the pineal gland (⧧). (Ref: Saldino RM, De Chiro G: Tentorial calcification. *Radiology* 1974; 111:207.)

FIG 1–85.—Calcification in the glomus of the choroid plexus of each lateral ventricle.

FIG 1–86.—Calcification in the glomus of the choroid plexus (boomerang configuration).

FIG 1–87.—Normal asymmetry of the calcified glomera of the choroid plexus. These cannot be reliably used for evidence of intracranial abnormality.

FIG 1–88.—Unilateral calcification of the glomus of the choroid plexus.

FIG 1–89.—Calcification of the internal carotid arteries.

FIG 1–90.—Calcification of the internal carotid arteries with very dense calcification in the lateral projection.

FIG 1–91.—Pituitary stones seen in lateral **(A)** and basal **(B)** projections in a 46-year-old man. These may be seen in asymptomatic patients as well as in those with hypopituitarism. (Ref: Taylor HC, et al: Pituitary stones and associated hypopituitarism. *JAMA* 1979; 242:751.)

FIG 1–92.—Large pituitary stone in a 20-year-old woman.

FIG 1–93.—Calcification in the dentate nucleus of the cerebellum. This form of calcification is not necessarily of clinical significance and may be physiologic.

FIG 1–94.—Idiopathic calcification of the basal ganglia may be familial and unassociated with other disease.

FIG 1–95.—Closing metopic suture mistaken for a fracture in a 1½-year-old boy. Closure occurs last in the cephalic end of the suture.

FIG 1–96.—Persistent metopic suture in a young adult. This suture may persist throughout life and be mistaken for a fracture.

FIG 1–97.—Persistent metopic suture, showing unusual serrations. The straight line is in the inner table, the serrated in the outer.

FIG 1–98.—Groove for the sagittal suture projected through the frontal bone, simulating a metopic suture.

FIG 1–99.—Unfused areas in the midline of the frontal bone (cranium bifidum occultum) in a 15-year-old child.

FIG 1–100.—Cranium bifidum occultum in a 9-month-old girl.

FIG 1–101.—Cranium bifidum occultum in a 14-month-old boy.

FIG 1–102.—Cranium bifidum occultum in a 28-year-old woman.

FIG 1–103.—*Top*, asymptomatic palpable developmental fossa in the frontal bone in an 8-month-old child. *Bottom*, at 5 years of age fossa is still present, essentially unchanged.

FIG 1–104.—Midline frontal accessory bone in an 11-month-old boy.

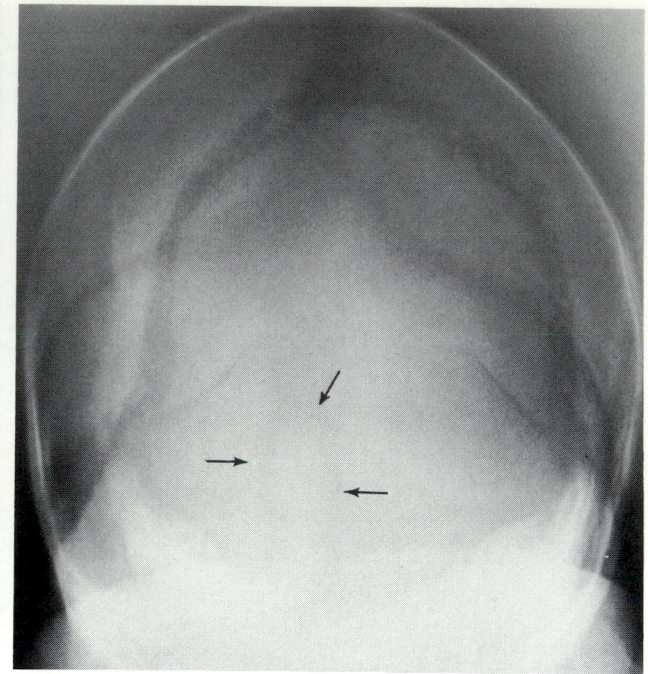

FIG 1–105.—Prominent nasofrontal suture, not to be mistaken for fracture. This suture may persist into adult life.

FIG 1–106.—Sclerosis of the nasofrontal suture, which might be mistaken for a meningioma of the anterior fossa.

FIG 1–107.—The nasofrontal suture in lateral projection.

FIG 1–108.—Large external occipital protuberance projected through frontal bone, simulating meningioma of the anterior fossa.

FIG 1–109.—Unusual scalloped appearance of the floor of the anterior fossa.

FIG 1–110.—Two examples of prominent frontal crests in children, simulating falx calcification.

FIG 1–111.—Vascular channel, simulating skull fracture. (Ref: Schunk H, Maruyama Y: Two vascular grooves of the external table of the skull which simulate fractures. *Acta Radiol* 1960; 54:186.)

FIG 1–112.—Unilateral serpentine vascular channels in the frontal bone.

FIG 1–113.—Vascular groove, simulating a fracture in a 1-year-old boy.

FIG 1–114.—Vascular channels above the frontal sinuses.

FIG 1–115.—Vascular channel of frontal bone, unusually well seen in lateral projection. (Courtesy of Dr. Wa'el M.A. Al-Bassam.)

FIG 1–116.—Three additional examples of frontal bone vascular grooves, which might be mistaken for fractures.

FIG 1–117.—Vascular groove in the frontal bone mistaken for a fracture. *Left*, plain film. *Right*, CT.

FIG 1–118.—Focal thickening of the inner table of the frontal bone.

FIG 1–119.—Nodular benign hyperostosis frontalis interna.

FIG 1–120.—Nebular hyperostosis frontalis interna.

FIG 1–121.—Diffuse benign hyperostosis of the frontal bone.

FIG 1–122.—Asymmetric localized hyperostosis frontalis interna in a 20-year-old woman.

FIG 1–123.—Asymmetric unilateral hyperostosis frontalis interna in a 28-year-old woman.

FIG 1–124.—Early asymmetric hyperostosis frontalis interna in a 35-year-old man. This entity is much less common in males.

FIG 1–125.—Hyperostosis frontalis interna with a simulated sequestrum.

FIG 1–126.—Hyperostosis frontalis interna with simulated doughnut lesion.

FIG 1–127.—Localized frontal calvarial osteoporotic thinning in an 84-year-old woman.

FIG 1–128.—Two neonates showing parietal fissures due to persistent strips of membranous bone matrix. These fissures disappear as the child matures and are often mistaken for fractures.

FIG 1–129.—Persistence of parietal fissure in a 1-year-old child, simulating a fracture.

FIG 1–130.—Unilateral intraparietal suture, which divides the parietal bone into an upper and lower segment. This suture may also occur bilaterally and extends from the coronal suture to the lambdoid suture. (Ref: Shapiro R: Anomalous parietal sutures and the bipartite parietal bone. *AJR* 1972; 115:569.)

FIG 1–131.—Unilateral intraparietal suture. When this suture is unilateral, the skull may be asymmetric, with the side harboring the intraparietal suture being larger than the opposite side, as in this case.

FIG 1–132.—Bilateral subsagittal sutures in a 1-year-old child.

FIG 1–133.—Unusual lucencies in the parietal bones crossing the midline, apparently representing a sagittal intrasutural bone, an incidental finding in an adult woman.

FIG 1–134.—Normal parietal foramina, which transmit the emissary veins of Santorini.

FIG 1–135.—Parietal emissary vascular channel. Note depression in the outer table at its point of exit.

FIG 1–136.—Parietal foramina. These congenital defects vary in size, but they are consistent in location and are often symmetric. They are not significant except in the differential diagnosis of cranial defects, including burr holes.

FIG 1–137.—Parietal foramina, showing some asymmetry.

FIG 1–138.—Paired parietal foramina, an unusual variant.

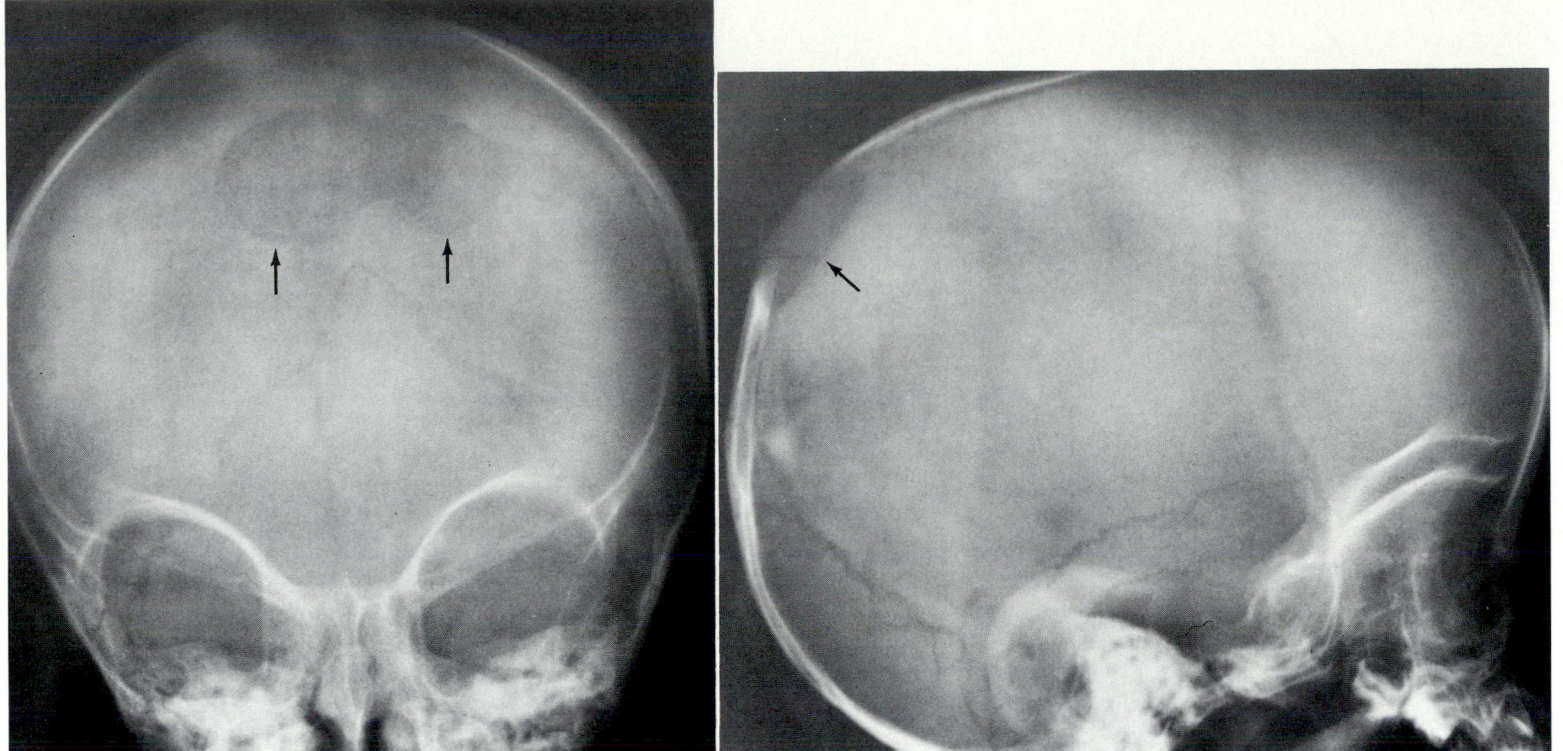

FIG 1–139.—Parietal foramina in a 15-month-old child without central dividing strip.

FIG 1–140.—Asymmetric and irregular parietal foramina.

FIG 1–141.—Unusual parietal foramina.

FIG 1–142.—Unusual venous vascular markings in parietal bone. This area frequently shows a striking vascular pattern.

FIG 1–143.—Localized area of thinning of external table at site of anterior fontanel. This should not be mistaken for erosion of the outer table.

FIG 1–144.—Parietal thinning, a manifestation of postmenopausal osteoporosis. The outer table is lost, with characteristic preservation of the inner table. Note also similar localized thinning of the frontal bone in the lateral projection. (Ref: Steinbach HL, Obata WG: The significance of thinning of the parietal bones. *AJR* 1957; 78:39.) Parietal thinning may rarely be unilateral. (Ref: Wilson AK: Thinness of parietal bones. *AJR* 1947; 58:724.)

FIG 1–145.—Combined parietal thinning and venous lakes and grooves in a 56-year-old woman.

FIG 1–146.—An 82-year-old man with parietal thinning. This entity is much less common in males.

FIG 1–147.—Hyperostosis generalisata and parietalis.

FIG 1–148.—Apparent malalignment of the parietal and occipital bones due to molding of labor, not to be mistaken for fracture (→). A cephalohematoma is present (↠).

FIG 1–149.— Unusual occipital configuration in the newborn due to the molding of labor.

FIG 1–150.—Occipital and parietal fissures due to persistent strips of membranous bone, a common finding in infants that may simulate fracture. The mendosal sutures are evident (↠).

FIG 1–151.—Fissures in an infant about foramen magnum similar to those of Figure 1–150.

FIG 1–152.—Persistant membranous fissures simulating fracture in an adolescent girl.

FIG 1–153.—Left, the synchondroses between the supraoccipital and exoccipital portions of the occipital bone in a 6-week-old child (→). The mendosal sutures are also seen (↠).

FIG 1–154.—Top, the mendosal suture (→) and synchondrosis between the supraoccipital and exoccipital portions of the occipital bone (↠) in lateral projection in a 1-month-old child.

FIG 1–156.—Appearance of the accessory supraoccipital ossicle in the lateral projection.

FIG 1–155.—Accessory ossicle of the supraoccipital bone (Kerckring's ossicle) in a normal infant. (Ref: Caffey J: On accessory ossicles of supraoccipital bone; some newly recognized roentgen features of normal infantile skull. *AJR* 1953; 70:401.)

FIG 1–158.—Occipital ossicle in the lateral projection.

FIG 1–157.—Unilateral ossicle of the supraoccipital bone.

FIG 1–159.—Irregular midline occipital ossicle in a 6-month-old girl.

FIG 1–160.—Persistence of an occipital ossicle in a 22-year-old man.

FIG 1–161.—Bathrocephaly in a 1-year-old child.

FIG 1–162.—Bathrocephaly in the adult, which may be confused with fracture.

FIG 1–163.—Bathrocephalic occiputs in adults.

FIG 1–164.— Bathrocephalic occiputs in adults.

FIG 1–165.— Normal, large interparietal bone in a 3-month-old child in frontal and lateral projections.

FIG 1–166.—Three examples of bifid interparietal bones (Inca bone). This should not be mistaken for a fracture. (Ref: Shapiro R, Robinson F: The os incae. *AJR* 1976; 127:469.)

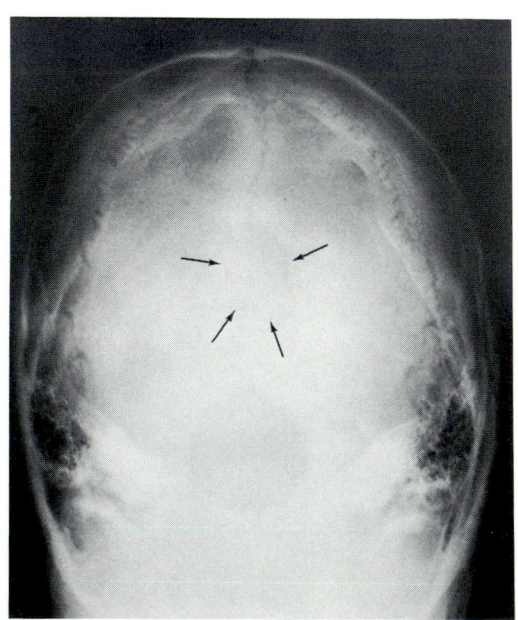

FIG 1–167.—Anterior fontanel bone seen in the occipital projection in a 14-year-old.

FIG 1–168.—Occipital flattening due to postural pressure, not to be confused with changes of craniostenosis.

FIG 1–169.—Two examples of how Inca bones may simulate fractures in the lateral projection.

FIG 1–170.—M-shaped Inca bone and occipital molding (breech head). This abnormal head shape is identified as a positive deformation associated with breech intrauterine position. It resolves during infancy with no residual impairment in most cases. (Ref. Haberkern CM, Smith DW, Jones KL: The "breech head" and its relevance. *Am J Dis Child* 1979; 133:154.)

FIG 1–171.—Cone-shaped interparietal bone.

FIG 1–172.—Rectangular interparietal bone in an adult.

FIG 1–173.—Paired, laterally placed interparietal bones.

FIG 1–174.—A small interparietal bone that has persisted into adult life.

FIG 1–175.—The superior median fissure of the occipital bone in a 21-month-old child, which should not be mistaken for fracture. Note also persistence of a strip of membranous bone simulating a fracture (→).

FIG 1–176.—Examples of asymmetric closure of the synchondrosis between the supraoccipital and exoccipital portions of the occipital bone. *Left*, 15-month-old infant. *Right*, 12-month-old infant. The open suture may be mistaken for fracture.

FIG 1–177.—Visualization of the inner and outer aspects of the lambdoidal suture, suggesting diastatic fracture.

FIG 1–178.—Persistent mendosal sutures in a 17-year-old boy.

FIG 1–179.—The mendosal suture in a 29-month-old child mistaken for a fracture in the frontal projection.

FIG 1–180.—Unilateral persistent mendosal suture in a 46-year-old man. **A,** frontal projection. **B,** occipital projection. **C,** lateral projection.

FIG 1–181.—PA and AP projections showing anomalous occipital suture, probably a remnant of the mendosal suture.

FIG 1–182.—Anomalous midline occipital suture (cerebellar synchondrosis). This is also a common site for fracture in small children, and the diagnosis of anomalous suture should be made with caution. *Left,* adult with sutural sclerosis evident. *Right,* child with no history of trauma. (Ref: Franken EA Jr: The midline occipital fissure: Diagnosis of fracture versus anatomic variants. *Radiology* 1969; 93:1043.)

FIG 1–183.—Two examples of asymmetric prominence of one occipitomastoid suture, suggesting fracture.

FIG 1–184.—Striking example of asymmetric prominence of one occipitomastoid suture, suggesting fracture, accentuated by slight rotation.

FIG 1–185.—The occipitomastoid sutures in frontal projections.

FIG 1–186.—Sutural bone in the occipitomastoid suture.

FIG 1–187.—Defects in the lambdoid suture, presumably representing persistent mastoid fontanels. The patient did not have neurofibromatosis.

FIG 1–188.—A portion of the sagittal suture seen through the occipital bone, simulating a fracture.

FIG 1–189.—The metopic suture may be seen in Towne projection and confused with a fracture. Note its continuation across the outline of the foramen magnum.

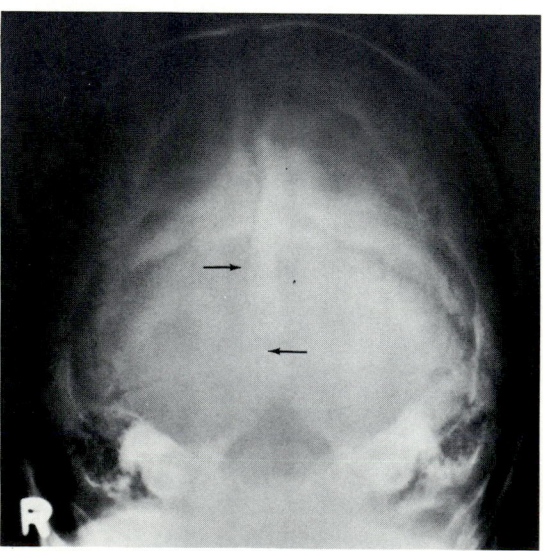

FIG 1–190.—Metopic suture, simulating occipital fracture in a 22-month-old child. Note lack of sutural serrations.

FIG 1–191.—Examples of occipital emissary channels.

FIG 1–192.—Two examples of the foramen for the occipital emissary vein, the in-ioendineal canal. This is a midline structure in contrast to the venous lakes, which are seen on both sides of the midline. (Ref: O'Rahilly R: Anomalous occipital apertures. *Arch Pathol* 1952; 53:509.)

FIG 1–193.—An unusual occipital emissary vein immediately above the foramen magnum.

FIG 1–194.—Midline vascular channel (←). Occipital venous lakes are also present (⫮).

FIG 1–195.—Occipital pacchionian impression.

FIG 1–196.—*Left,* occipital pacchionian impression (←). Note draining vein (↔). *Right,* CT confirmation.
(Ref: Skully RD, Mark EJ, McNeely BV: Case 42-1984: Pacchionian granulation. *N Engl J Med* 1984; 322:1036.)

FIG 1–197.—Occipital venous lakes. These structures vary widely in number and appearance. They are usually seen near the midline of the occipital bone, most commonly in older individuals. These lakes lie in the diploic space and are of no clinical significance. (From Keats TE: Four normal anatomic variations of importance to radiologists. *AJR* 1957; 78:89. Used by permission.) There is evidence that identical occipital radiolucencies may be the product of ectopic neural tissue. These are similarly without clinical significance. (Ref: Goldring S, et al: Ectopic neural tissue of the occipital bone. *J Neurosurg* 1964; 21:479.)

FIG 1–198.—Large midline occipital venous lake.

FIG 1–199.—Venous lakes may often be seen in the diploic space in the lateral projection.

FIG 1–200.—Similar occipital radiolucencies with CT demonstration.

FIG 1–201.—Other variations of occipital venous lakes.

FIG 1–202.—Development of occipital venous lake. The film on the right was exposed 16 years after the film on the left.

FIG 1–203.—Occipital venous lake with prominent draining venous channel.

FIG 1–204.— Normal unilateral prominence of the groove for the transverse venous sinus.

FIG 1–205.—The transverse sinuses seen on end, evidenced as lucencies in the mastoids.

FIG 1–206.—Prominent transverse venous sinuses, producing striking radiolucency in the lateral projection.

FIG 1–207.—Occipital midline radiolucency, probably representing a closure defect. There were no associated clinical findings.

FIG 1–208.—Localized thickening of the occipital bone, a normal variant.

FIG 1–209.—Striking appearance of occipital region produced by venous sinuses and normal lucency of the occipital bones.

FIG 1–210.—The occipital bone may have a variety of symmetric or asymmetric areas of thinning near the midline, which may simulate erosion of the inner table. Some of them relate to the configuration of the transverse venous sinuses. It is important that the innocence of these variants be recognized. The crossed arrows (⧧) indicate the venous sinuses.

FIG 1–211.—Developmental thinning of the occipital bone **(A)** proved by CT. The defect contains normal brain **(B).** (From Haden MA, Keats TE: The anatomic basis for localized occipital thinning: A normal anatomic variant. *Skeletal Radiol* 1982; 8:221. Used by permission.)

FIG 1–212.—Additional examples of occipital thinning. Note similarity to changes of erosion of inner table.

FIG 1–213.—Asymmetric occipital thinning below the torcula in 28-year-old woman.

FIG 1–214.—Occipital thinning near midline.

FIG 1–215.—Small discrete area of occipital thinning.

FIG 1–216.—Symmetric occipital thinning above the torcula in a 26-year-old woman. It has been suggested that the lucencies in this location may coincide with the occipital poles, best observed in patients with thin cranial vaults. (Ref: Newton TH, Potts DG: *Radiology of the Skull and Brain.* St Louis, CV Mosby Co, 1971, vol 1, p 157.)

FIG 1–217.—Symmetric areas of occipital thinning, simulating a pneumoencephalogram.

FIG 1–218.—Occipital thinning seen in lateral projection above the transverse sinuses. Note apparent loss of the inner table of the calvarium.

FIG 1–219.—Large asymmetric occipital thinning in a 43-year-old woman.

FIG 1–220.— Normal asymmetry of the condyloid canals (←). A small ossicle is present in the right canal. Note also the normal irregularity of the posterior margin of the foramen magnum (⧺). (Ref: Gathier JC, Bruyn GW: The so-called condyloid foramen in the half-axial view. *AJR* 1969; 107:515.)

FIG 1–221.—Asymmetric condyloid fossae with a large fossa on the patient's left (←). The condyloid canal is seen within the fossa (⧺).

FIG 1–222.—Prominent external occipital protuberance producing a midline density in the half-axial projection.

FIG 1–223.—Huge external occipital protuberance.

FIG 1–224.—Prominent external occipital protuberance with adjacent calcification in the ligamentum nuchae.

FIG 1–225.—Radiolucency produced by base of the external occipital protuberance.

FIG 1–226.—Unusual appearance produced by superimposition of external occipital protuberance and confluence of the venous sinuses.

FIG 1–227.—Simulated abnormality of foramen magnum, produced by superimposed projection of benign hyperostosis of the internal surface of frontal bone.

FIG 1–228.—Two examples of normal irregularities of the margins of the foramen magnum.

FIG 1–229.—Paracondylar process. This cone-shaped bony structure projects down from the lateral aspect of the occipital condyle toward the transverse process of C-1. It may be unilateral or bilateral. **A,** lateral projection. **B** and **C,** tomograms. (Ref: Shapiro R, Robinson F: Anomalies of the craniovertebral border. *AJR* 1976; 127:281.)

FIG 1–230.—The squamoparietal suture in an 8-month-old should not be mistaken for fracture (see Fig 1–47).

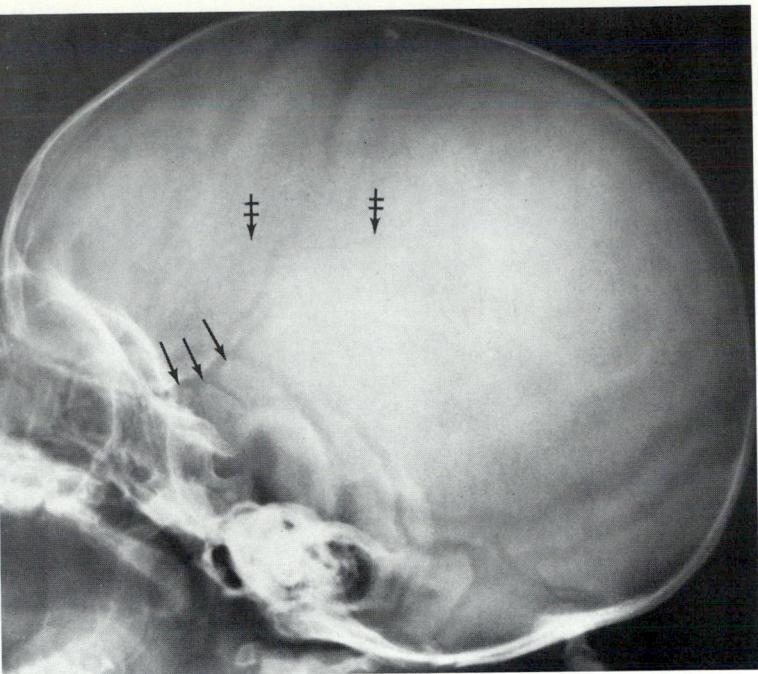

FIG 1–231.—Vascular grooves in the temporal bone seen through the sphenoid sinus, simulating fractures.

FIG 1–232.—Skull of 3-month-old infant, showing wormian bones in the anterior end of the squamosal suture (←). Note also the vascular groove in the parietal bone that simulates fracture (⫢). The skull is rotated on its vertical axis, and the groove is projected across the coronal sutures.

FIG 1–233.—Two examples of grooves for the middle temporal artery, simulating fracture. (Ref: Schunk H, Maruyama Y: Two vascular grooves of the external table of the skull that simulate fractures. *Acta Radiol* 1960; 54:186.)

FIG 1–234.—Two examples of vascular grooves in the temporal bone, simulating fractures. (Ref: Allen WE, et al: Pitfalls in the evaluation of skull trauma. *Radiol Clin North Am* 1973; 11:479.)

FIG 1–235.—Additional examples of vascular grooves that may be mistaken for fractures.

FIG 1–236.—Convolutional impressions. The scalloping of the inner table of the middle cranial fossa is normal in adult skulls. (Ref: Lane B: Erosions of the skull. *Radiol Clin North Am* 1974; 12:257.)

FIG 1–237.—Two examples of temporal sutural sclerosis, simulating suprasellar calcification.

FIG 1–238.—Focal area of sclerosis in the squamosal suture in a 76-year-old woman.

FIG 1–239.—Exaggeration of the normal lucency of the squamosal portion of the temporal bone.

FIG 1–240.—Temporal thinning in Stenver's projection, simulating destruction of the calvarium.

FIG 1–241.—Isolated hyperostosis interna of the temporal bones.

FIG 1–242.—Large antrum, simulating destructive lesion.

FIG 1–243.—Air in the external auditory canal, seen as discrete radiolucency.

FIG 1–244.—Mastoid emissary vein seen unilaterally in Towne's projection (←). Note the prominent condyloid fossa on the opposite side (⫛).

FIG 1–245.—Large mastoid antra, which might be mistaken for cholesteatomas. (Ref: Tillitt R, et al: The large mastoid antrum. *Radiology* 1970; 94:619.)

FIG 1–246.—**A,** an example of unusually marked pneumatization of the mastoids. **B,** detailed view of the mastoid air cells.

FIG 1–247.—Extremely marked pneumatization of the mastoid.

FIG 1–248.—*Left,* asymmetric development of the mastoids in a 5-year-old child, with marked overdevelopment on the patient's right side. Note lucency in the midline of the occipital bone, which represents a normal variant (see Fig 1–211). *Right,* detailed view of the right mastoid.

FIG 1–249.—Large asymmetric mastoid air cell, which might be mistaken for an area of bone destruction.

FIG 1–250.—Large mastoid air cell below emissary vein, simulating an area of bone destruction.

FIG 1–251.—Large mastoid emissary vein.

FIG 1–252.—Large mastoid emissary vein.

FIG 1–253.—Sigmoid sinus (←) and mastoid emissary vein (⧧).

FIG 1–254.—Normal asymmetry in height of the petrous ridges. This entity may be associated occasionally with trigeminal neuralgia. (Ref: Obrador S, et al: Trigeminal neuralgia secondary to asymmetry of the petrous bone. *J Neurosurg* 1970; 33:596.)

FIG 1–255.—Two examples of normal asymmetry in height and configuration of the petrous ridges.

FIG 1–256.—Large mastoid air cells at the petrous tips, simulating the changes of acoustic neuroma. (Ref: Dubois PJ, Roub LW: Giant air cell of petrous apex. *Radiology* 1978; 129:103.)

FIG 1–257.—Stenver's projection of the petrous tips of the case illustrated in Figure 1–256.

FIG 1–258.—Pneumatization of one petrous tip simulating enlargement of the internal auditory meatus.

FIG 1–259.—Apparent destruction of the petrous tips due to pneumatization.

FIG 1–260.—Asymmetric pneumatization of the petrous ridges.

FIG 1-261.—Dense nodular form of calcification of the petroclinoid ligament, simulating asymmetric development of one petrous bone, with dense portion seen in lateral projection.

FIG 1-262.—The os supra petrosum of Meckel (see Fig 1-73).

FIG 1-263.—*Left,* small, rounded bony knob on the superior margin of the petrous bones. This finding is usually unilateral but may be bilateral as in this case. (Ref: Shapiro R: An interesting normal variant of the temporal bone. *Radiology* 1978; 128:354). *Right,* bony ring-like configuration of the petrous tip.

FIG 1–264.—Variation in development of the petrous ridges, producing an anomalous "foramen" on one side. **A,** plain film. **B,** laminagram.

FIG 1–265.—"Fish-mouth" internal auditory meatus by tomography, one of the normal variations in configuration.

FIG 1–266.—Two examples of normal asymmetry of configuration of the internal auditory canals. (Ref: Fraser RA, Carter BL: Unilateral dilatation of the internal auditory canal. *Neuroradiology* 1975; 9:227.)

FIG 1−267.—Normal asymmetry of the lesser wings of the sphenoid. Note arching of the wing on the left.

FIG 1−268.—Asymmetry of the lesser wings of the sphenoid in a normal individual, simulating bone destruction on the right (←). Note also the normal asymmetry of the superior orbital fissures (⇜). (Ref: Shapiro R, Robinson F: Alterations of the sphenoidal fissure produced by local and systemic processes. *AJR* 1967; 101:814.)

FIG 1−269.—Asymmetry of the lesser wings of the sphenoid (←) and superior orbital fissures (⇜).

FIG 1−270.—Marked asymmetry of the superior orbital fissures.

FIG 1–271.—Four additional examples of normal variation and asymmetry of the lesser wings of the sphenoid.

FIG 1–272.—Simulated fracture of the lesser wing of the sphenoid by anatomic variation not present on opposite side. **A,** plain film. **B,** tomogram.

FIG 1–273.—Developmental spurs from the lesser wings of the sphenoid.

FIG 1–274.—Slight rotation of the head and the superimposition of a prominent external occipital protuberance, appearing on the right, simulating the changes of a sphenoid wing meningioma.

FIG 1–275.—Two examples of pneumatization of the anterior clinoid processes, simulating enlargement of the optic foramina.

FIG 1–276.—Asymmetric pneumatization of the anterior clinoid processes, simulating abnormality of the optic canals.

FIG 1–277.—Lateral extension of sphenoidal sinus air cell into the greater wing of the sphenoid, simulating a destructive lesion.

FIG 1–278.—Lateral strut of the lesser wing of the sphenoid, simulating changes of a meningioma.

FIG 1–279.—The pterion, which may simulate meningioma of the planum sphenoidale.

FIG 1–280.—The nonunited ossification center of the presphenoid bone that might be mistaken for evidence of a meningioma. *Left,* separate, well-corticated ossicle *(arrow)* posterior and superior to the anterior clinoid. *Right,* AP tomogram showing separate center at the anterior clinoid process. The anterior clinoids are superior and the inferior clinoids are inferior. (From Ratner LM, Quencer RM: Nonunited ossification center of the presphenoid bone: Pseudomeningioma. *AJR* 1983; 143:503–506. Used by permission.)

FIG 1–281.—The coronal suture, seen in the base view, simulating a fracture.

FIG 1–282.—The sagittal suture, seen in the base view, simulating a fracture.

FIG 1–283.—The occipitomastoid sutures in the basal views of the skull.

FIG 1–284.—The squamosal suture in the base view.

FIG 1–285.—Vascular groove in the vertex of the skull, simulating a basal skull fracture.

FIG 1–286.—The synchondrosis between the basisphenoid and basiocciput in a 2-year-old boy. This suture normally closes near puberty but may persist until the 20th year. It is at times mistaken for fracture.

FIG 1–287.—The basisphenoid-basiocciput synchondrosis in a 5-year-old girl by laminagraphy.

FIG 1–288.—The sphenofrontal suture in a 3-month-old child.

FIG 1–289.—The sphenofrontal suture (←) and the sphenotemporal sutures (⫢) in an 18-month-old child. Note also the basisphenoid-basiocciput synchondrosis (⫣).

FIG 1–290.—The unfused planum sphenoidale (←), simulating a fracture. This is a developmental variation. In fractures, the anterior fragment of the planum is depressed, as compared with this variation in which the planum is superior to the chiasmatic sulcus (⧺). (Ref: Smith TR, Kier EL: The unfused planum sphenoidale: Differentiation from fracture. *Radiology* 1971; 98:305.)

FIG 1–291.—Normal asymmetry of the basal foramina. (Ref: Shapiro R, Robinson F: The foramina of the middle fossa: A phylogenetic, anatomic and pathologic study. *AJR* 1967; 101:779.)

FIG 1–292.—An example of striking asymmetry of the basal foramina. The foramen ovale (←) and the foramen spinosum (⧺) are confluent on the patient's right, simulating destruction of the base of the skull. (Ref: Newton TH, Potts DG: *Radiology of the Skull and Brain.* St Louis, Mosby-Year Book, 1971, vol 1, p 306.)

FIG 1–293.—Foramen ovale with a petroalar bar. (Ref: Newton TH, Potts DG: *Radiology of the Skull and Brain.* St Louis, Mosby-Year Book, 1971, vol 1, p 310.)

FIG 1–294.—Normal asymmetry of the foramina ovalea, also seen in Waters projection on the right.

FIG 1–295.—Marked asymmetric development of the foramina ovalea.

FIG 1–296.—Very large jugular foramina with striking prominence on the left (←). Note the unusual shadow in the nasopharynx due to the epiglottis (⫣).

FIG 1–297.—Large carotid foramen seen unilaterally.

FIG 1–298.—Simulated fossae produced by the rectus capitis muscle attachments.

FIG 1–299.—The foramen ovale with a pterygospinous bar. (Ref: Newton TH, Potts DG: *Radiology of the Skull and Brain*. St Louis, CV Mosby Co, 1971, vol 1, p 307.)

FIG 1–300.—The junction of the frontal and ethmoid bones in a 3-month-old child might be mistaken for a fracture.

FIG 1–301.—A large sphenoidal air cell, simulating an enlarged basal foramen.

FIG 1–302.—Pneumatization of the pterygoid bones producing unusual radiolucency in the base of the skull.

FIG 1–303.—Normal asymmetry of foramina rotunda seen in Caldwell's *(left)* and asymmetry of the infraorbital foramina seen in Waters projection *(right)*.

FIG 1–304.—Pneumatization of the clinoid processes may produce spurious foramen-like shadows in the basal view.

FIG 1–305.—The nasolacrimal canals.

FIG 1–306.—Soft tissue masses seen in the nasopharyngeal air shadow, representing large pharyngeal tonsils.

FIG 1–307.—The uvula seen in the nasopharyngeal air shadow.

FIG 1–308.—Large occipital condyles. *Left*, AP projection. *Center*, lateral projection. *Right*, tomogram.

FIG 1–309.—Unfused anterior arch of C-1 in basal view of the skull.

FIG 1–310.—Shadow of the folded ear, simulating suprasellar calcification.

FIG 1–311.—The intersphenoidal synchondrosis in a newborn. This entity should not be mistaken for a fracture, a persistent basipharyngeal canal, or the spheno-occipital synchondrosis. It has no pathologic significance and usually disappears by 3 years of age. (Ref: Shopfner CE, et al: The intersphenoid synchondrosis. *AJR* 1968; 104:184.)

FIG 1–312.—Partially obliterated intersphenoidal synchondrosis in a 2-year-old child.

FIG 1–313.—Obliterated intersphenoidal synchondrosis in an adult.

FIG 1–314.—The basipharyngeal canal in a 10-year-old boy.

FIG 1–315.—Large normal tuberculum sellae.

FIG 1–316.—Well-defined middle clinoid process.

FIG 1–317.—Additional examples of prominent middle clinoid processes.

FIG 1–318.—Bridging of the sella due to calcification of the interclinoid ligaments.

FIG 1–319.—Bridging of the sella in a 5½-month-old child.

FIG 1–320.—Ligamentous calcification between the posterior and middle clinoid processes.

FIG 1–321.—The sellar spine, an anatomic variant of no clinical significance. (From: Dietemann JL, et al: Anatomy and radiology of the sellar spine. *Neuroradiology* 1981; 21:5. Used by permission.)

FIG 1–322.—Bridging between the anterior and middle clinoid processes.

FIG 1–323.—Well-defined tuberculum sellae.

FIG 1–324.—Very large clinoid processes, producing apparent bridging of the sella.

FIG 1–325.—Pneumatization of the planum sphenoidale, producing unusual appearance.

FIG 1–326.—Two examples of the radiolucency of a thin dorsum sellae, simulating a destructive process.

FIG 1–327.—Mushroom configuration of the posterior clinoid processes.

FIG 1–328.—Unusual appearance of the dorsum sellae due to heavy calcification of the petroclinoid ligament.

FIG 1–329.—Normal variations in the shape of the sella turcica. Tiny sellae may normally be seen. (Ref: Swanson HA, Du Boulay G: Borderline variants of the normal pituitary fossa. *Br J Radiol* 1975; 48:366.)

FIG 1–330.—Normal variations in the shape of the sella turcica. **A,** the small sella. **B,** the shallow sella.

FIG 1–331.—Double floor of the sella, produced by filming in less than true lateral projection.

FIG 1–332.—Double floor of the sella, simulated by the carotid groove.

FIG 1–333.—Double floor of the sella due to inclination of the floor of the sella. (Ref: Tenner MS, Weitzman I Jr: Pitfalls in the diagnosis of erosive changes in the expanding lesions of the pituitary fossa. *Radiology* 1980; 137:393.)

FIG 1–334.—Double floor of the sella due to unequal sphenoid sinus development. **A,** lateral projection. **B,** AP tomogram. (Ref: Bruneton JN, et al: Normal variants of the sella turcica. *Radiology* 1979; 131:99.)

FIG 1–335.—Normal variation of the sella turcica. Note the small bridged sella.

FIG 1–336.—Normal variations of the sella turcica. **A,** hidden anterior clinoid processes due to pneumatization. **B,** extensive pneumatization of the clinoid processes and dorsum sellae.

FIG 1–337.—Extensive pneumatization of the dorsum sellae, simulating erosion.

Chapter 2

The Facial Bones

FIG 2–1.—Normal asymmetry of the lesser wings of the sphenoid.

FIG 2–2.—Pneumatization of the anterior clinoid processes, simulating enlargement of the optic canals.

FIG 2–3.—Bilateral congenital absence of the orbital processes of the zygoma.

FIG 2–4.—Simulated destruction of the lateral wall of the orbit, resulting from through-projection of the transverse venous sinus.

FIG 2–5.—The anterior clinoid processes superimposed on the superior orbital fissures.

FIG 2–6.—Simulated fracture through zygomaticofrontal suture, produced by a slight rotation of the head.

FIG 2–7.—Unusual appearance produced by extension of a sphenoidal air cell into the greater wing of the sphenoid.

FIG 2–8.—Ethmoidal air cell, simulating trauma in a patient with facial trauma. **A,** plain film. **B,** tomogram.

FIG 2–9.—Asymmetric supraorbital foramina. This may be confused with a localized destruction of the orbital rim.

FIG 2–10.—Asymmetric supraorbital foramina.

FIG 2–11.—Two examples of normal asymmetry of the superior orbital fissures.

FIG 2–12.—Normal asymmetry of the superior orbital fissures (←). Note also the asymmetric density of the sphenoidal wings and the apparent loss of the superior medial aspect of the right orbital rim (⊬).

FIG 2–13.—Factitial increased density of the left orbit due to a slight rotation of the head and a prominent superimposed external occipital protuberance.

FIG 2–14.—Periglobal fat, simulating air in the orbits (→). Note also the shadow of the closed eyelids (⇸).

FIG 2–15.—The shadow of the eyelid seen unilaterally.

FIG 2–16.—The edge of the superior orbital fissure, not to be mistaken for calcification in the globe.

FIG 2–17.—Two examples of the infraorbital groove, simulating a fracture of the floor of the orbit. The patient on the right has sinusitis.

FIG 2–18.—Hypoplasia of both antra, simulating sinus disease.

FIG 2–19.—Hypoplasia of the maxillary antrum, simulating sinus disease.

FIG 2–20.—Two examples of unilateral hypoplasia of the maxillary antrum. This condition may be associated with asymmetry of the superior orbital fissures. (Ref: Bassiouny A, et al: Maxillary sinus hypoplasia and superior orbital fissure asymmetry. *Laryngoscope* 1982; 92:441.)

FIG 2–21.—Hypoplasia of the maxillary antrum. Note enlargement of the orbit on the same side, a finding that frequently accompanies hypoplasia of the antrum. (Ref: Bierny JP, Dryden R: Orbital enlargement secondary to paranasal sinus hypoplasia. *AJR* 1977; 128:850.)

FIG 2–22.—Hypoplasia of the left maxillary antrum.

FIG 2–23.—Hypoplasia of the antrum on the left (←). Note also the lateral extension of the right sphenoid sinus, producing an apparent loculation of the antrum (⧧).

FIG 2–24.—Unusual development of the maxillary antra. **A,** plain film. The right antrum is huge and extends far laterally. The left antrum contains at least two loculi, the medial one being deeper and more lucent than the lateral. **B,** laminagram.

FIG 2–25.—Compartmented antra in a patient with sinusitis.

FIG 2–26.—Four examples of apparent loculation of the antra, produced by lateral extension of sphenoidal sinus air cells.

FIG 2–27.—Localized bony excrescence in roof of antrum probably due to incomplete aeration around the infraorbital canal and foramen.

FIG 2–28.—Localized bony thickening of the lateral wall of the maxillary antrum.

FIG 2–29.—Localized bony excrescence in the floor of the maxillary antrum.

FIG 2–30.—Simulated fractures of the lateral wall of the maxillary antrum, produced by the posterior superior alveolar canal. (Ref: Chuang VP, Vines FS: Roentgenology of the posterior superior alveolar foramina and canals. *AJR* 1973; 118:426.)

FIG 2–31.—The nares superimposed on the antra, simulating polyps.

FIG 2–32.—The upper lip superimposed on the antra, simulating retention cysts.

FIG 2–33.—Two examples of simulated tumor of the antrum, produced by superimposition of the turbinates on the coronoid process of the mandible. (Ref: Sistrom CL, Keats TE, Johnson CM III: The anatomic basis of the pseudotumor of the nasal cavity. *AJR* 1986; 147:782.)

FIG 2–34.—The coronoid process of the mandible, illustrating the mechanism of production of the pseudotumor shown in Figure 2–33.

FIG 2–35.—The coronoid process of the mandible in the brow-up projection, simulating an air-fluid level in the maxillary antrum.

FIG 2–36.—Overdevelopment of the frontal sinuses without associated disease.

FIG 2–37.—Unilateral development of the frontal sinuses.

FIG 2–38.—Unusual variation in pneumatization of the frontal sinus with an anomalous air cell, simulating an intradiploic epidermoid.

FIG 2–39.—Incomplete pneumatization of the anterior wall of the frontal sinus, producing a mass effect in the sinus.

FIG 2–40.—Incomplete aeration of the frontal sinus, producing shadowing of the frontal sinuses. Osseous shadows are evident in the lateral projection *(arrow)*.

FIG 2–41.—Uneven aeration of the frontal sinuses due to irregularity of the posterior wall.

FIG 2–42.—Marked cephalad extension of the frontal sinus.

FIG 2–43.—Large lateral locule of the frontal sinus.

FIG 2–44.—Marked lateral extension of the frontal sinus.

FIG 2–45.—Marked posterior extension of the frontal sinuses.

FIG 2–46.—Discrete cellule within the frontal sinus, probably arising from an ethmoidal air cell.

FIG 2–47.—Two examples of factitial clouding of the frontal sinus, produced by superimposition of a large external occipital protuberance.

FIG 2–48.—Sclerosis of the nasofrontal suture.

FIG 2–49.—A sclerotic lambdoidal suture superimposed on the edge of the frontal sinus, mistaken for osteomyelitis.

FIG 2–50.—Bowed central septum of the frontal sinus.

FIG 2–51.—Remarkable overdevelopment of the ethmoidal air cells, with extension into the floor of the anterior fossa.

FIG 2–52.—Marked pneumatization of the crista galli.

FIG 2–53.—Less marked pneumatization of the crista galli (←). The arrows below (⧸⧸) indicate the foramina rotunda.

FIG 2–55.—Laminagram of the ethmoidal region, showing asymmetric development of the foramina rotunda with poor definition of the lateral aspect of one of the foramina.

FIG 2–54.—An anomalous ethmoidal air cell in the floor of the orbit.

FIG 2–56.—Ethmoidal cell extending into the sphenoid sinus.

FIG 2–57.—Ethmoidal cell extending into a nonaerated sphenoid sinus, resulting in a mass effect in the sphenoid sinus. **A,** plain film. **B,** tomogram.

FIG 2–58.—Apparent air-fluid level in the sphenoid sinus produced by incomplete aeration. The film was made upright, but not brow-up.

FIG 2–59.—*Top,* simulated air-fluid level in the sphenoid sinus produced by the zygomatic arch. *Bottom,* heavier exposure shows bony detail to better advantage. (Ref: Swenson WE: Zygomatic arch simulating an air-fluid level in the sphenoid sinus. *Br J Radiol* 1988; 61:518.)

FIG 2–60.—Pneumatization of the pterygoid plates.

FIG 2–61.—Unusual appearance produced by extension of a sphenoidal air cell into the greater wing of the sphenoid. (Ref: Yune HY, et al: Normal variations and lesions of the sphenoid sinus. *AJR* 1975; 124:129.)

FIG 2–62.—Marked lateral and inferior extensions of the sphenoid sinuses.

FIG 2–63.—Unusually marked lateral extension of the sphenoid sinuses. (Ref: Kattan KR, Potter GY: Lateral extension of sphenoid sinuses. *Med Radiogr Photogr* 1983; 59:9.)

FIG 2–64.—The zygomaticotemporal foramen (Hyrtl's foramen). (Ref: Yanagisawa E, Smith HW: Normal radiographic anatomy of the paranasal sinuses. *Otolaryngol Clin North Am* 1973; 6:434.)

FIG 2–65.—Laminagram of the zygomatic arch showing the suture between the zygomatic bone and the zygomatic process of the temporal bone. This suture may be confused with a fracture line.

FIG 2–66.— The suture between the zygomatic bone and the zygomatic process of the temporal bone seen in oblique projection, simulating a fracture.

FIG 2–67.—Simulated fracture of the zygomatic arch, produced by overlapping shadows of the base and arch of the bone.

FIG 2–68.—The zygomaxillary suture in a 6-year-old boy, simulating a fracture.

FIG 2–69.—Air cell in the zygomatic arch.

FIG 2–70.—Pneumatization of the condylar fossa **(A),** which might be mistaken for arthritic change. Compare with opposite side **(B).**

FIG 2–71.—Spur-like insertion of the temporomandibular ligament.

FIG 2–72.—Overlapping shadow of the tongue, simulating fracture of the condyle of the mandible. (Courtesy of Dr. Rahmat O. Kashef.)

FIG 2–73.—A, pharyngeal air shadow over the base of the tongue superimposed on the mandible simulates a fracture. B, Panorex film made at same session shows that no fracture is present.

FIG 2–74.—Two examples of how the pharyngeal air shadows may simulate a fracture of the mandible.

FIG 2–75.—Superimposition of the airway, producing an apparent fracture of the mandibular condyle.

FIG 2–76.—The mandibular canal, simulating calcification in soft tissues.

FIG 2–77.—Simulated fractures of the coronoid processes produced by superimposition of the lateral pterygoid plates.

FIG 2–78.—Irregularity of the mandibular angles due to the insertion of the masseter muscles.

FIG 2–80.—Entry point of the mandibular nerve, simulating fracture of the mandible.

FIG 2–79.—Prominent mandibular angles, simulating exostoses.

FIG 2–81.—**A,** coronoid process of the mandible mistaken for an osteoma. **B,** basal view in another patient illustrates the origin of the density seen in **A.**

FIG 2–82.—Very large geniohyoid tubercle.

FIG 2–83.—The normal mental foramina.

FIG 2–84.—The mental foramen (→). Note how it can be mistaken for an apical abscess (⇸).

FIG 2–85.— The dental crypt of a partially erupted molar should not be mistaken for an apical abscess.

FIG 2–86.—Crypts for the third molars in a 9-year-old child that should not be mistaken for dental cysts.

FIG 2–87.—Prominent mandibular canals.

FIG 2–88.—The earlobes visualized by Panorex radiography.

FIG 2–89.—The normal nasal bone. Note the nasomaxillary suture (→) and the grooves for the nasociliary nerves (↠). No grooves should cross the nasal bridge. (Ref: de Lacey GJ, et al: The radiology of nasal injuries: Problems of interpretation and clinical relevance. *Br J Radiol* 1977; 50:412.)

FIG 2–90.—Hypoplasia of the nasal bone.

FIG 2–91.—Pneumatized middle turbinates (concha bullosa).

FIG 2–92.—Turbinate air stripes.

FIG 2–93.—*Top*, Waters' projection suggesting a mass in the nasal passage produced by a large inferior turbinate. *Bottom*, the nature of the mass effect is evident in the Caldwell projection.

Chapter 3

The Spine

FIG 3–1.—The neural canal in the infant is proportionately larger than that in the adult. This difference is often overlooked in the infant and may be misinterpreted as a manifestation of pathologic expansion of the spinal canal. **A** and **B,** a 4-month-old infant. **C** and **D,** an 18-year-old man.

FIG 3–2.—Apparent enlargement of the cervical spinal canal in a neonate due to flexion of the head at the time of filming and lordotic projection.

FIG 3–3.—Enlargement of the cervical canal with no evidence of cervical cord lesions in normal children. **A** and **B,** plain films showing marked enlargement of cervical canal. **C** and **D,** myelograms showing large dural sac with normal cord. The same phenomenon may also be seen in the thoracic spine (see Fig 3–252). (Ref: Yousefzadeh DK, et al: Normal sagittal diameter and variation in the pediatric cervical spine. *Radiology* 1982; 144:319.)

FIG 3–4.—Large cervical canal in a healthy 4 ½-year-old girl (see Figs 3–3 and 3–286).

FIG 3–5.—Simulated craniovertebral dislocation resulting from slight tilting of the head at the time of filming. *Right*, tomogram shows normal relationships of C-1 to base of skull.

FIG 3–6.—Complete incorporation of C-1 into the base of the skull (assimilation of the atlas).

FIG 3–7.—Partial incorporation of C-1 into the base of the skull. Note incomplete segmentation of C2–3 as well.

FIG 3–8.—Partial incorporation of C-1 into the base of the skull to a lesser degree than that pictured in Figure 3–7. Note also similar incomplete segmentation of C2–3.

FIG 3–9.—Occipital vertebra. The third condyle (←). A unilateral paracondylar process is present, which articulates with the transverse process of the atlas (⊬). (Ref: Lombardi G: The occipital vertebra. *AJR* 1961; 86:260.)

FIG 3–10.—Hypoplastic odontoid (←). There is a spina bifida occulta of C-2 producing an apparent cleft in the odontoid (↔).

FIG 3–11.—A smaller third occipital condyle.

FIG 3–12.—Anomalous articulation between the posterior arch of C-1 and the base of the skull.

FIG 3–13.—A second example of anomalous articulation between the posterior arch of C–1 and the base of the skull.

FIG 3–14.—Attempt to form an anomalous articulation between the posterior arch of C-1 and the base of the skull.

FIG 3–15.—Paracondylar process arising from the occipital bone (see Fig 1–229).

FIG 3–16.—Epitransverse process arises from the transverse process of the atlas and projects cranial toward the occipital condyle. It is a mirror image of the paracondylar process (see Fig 1–229). The epitransverse process may be unilateral or bilateral and may coexist with the paracondylar process. (Ref: Shapiro R, Robinson F: Anomalies of the craniovertebral border. *AJR* 1976; 127:281.)

FIG 3–17.—Bony spur arising from the base of the skull, simulating a neural arch (→). Note the arcuate foramina for the vertebral arteries (⇢).

FIG 3–18.—Two examples of accessory bony elements between the base of the skull and the neural arch of C-1.

FIG 3–19.—A, normal cleft in the neural arch of the atlas in a 1-year-old child. **B,** normal clefts in the neural arches of all the cervical vertebrae in an 11-month-old child. These neurocentral synchondroses may persist until the third to sixth years and may persist unilaterally for several months after the other side has closed. (Ref: Swischuk LE, et al: The dens-arch synchondroses vs. the hangman's fracture. *Pediatr Radiol* 1979; 8:100.)

FIG 3–20.—Incomplete closure of the neural arch of C-1 in a 2-year-old child. These normally close at 3 to 6 years of age.

FIG 3–21.—Complete absence of the posterior neural arch of C-1. (Ref: Dalinka MK, et al: Congenital absence of the posterior arch of the atlas. *Radiology* 1972; 103:581.)

FIG 3–22.—Two examples of absence of posterior arch of C-1. Note marked overgrowth of the spinous process of C-2.

FIG 3–23.—Absence of the laminae of C-1. (Ref: Logan WW, Stuard ID: Absent posterior arch of the atlas. *AJR* 1973; 118:431.) This entity is not necessarily innocent and may be associated with instability. (Ref: Schultze P, Bourman R: Absence of the posterior arch of the atlas. *AJR* 1982; 134:178.)

FIG 3–24.—Two examples of incomplete formation of the posterior neural arch of C-1.

FIG 3–25.—Incomplete formation of the neural arch of C-1 with fragment seen in lateral projection **(A)** and in Towne projection **(B)**.

FIG 3–26.—Incomplete formation of the posterior arch of C-1 with spina bifida occulta seen in the frontal projection (→).

FIG 3–27.—*Left,* incomplete development of the neural arch of C-1 simulating a fracture. *Right,* CT shows partial formation on the right side of the neural arch.

FIG 3–28.—Failure of fusion of the posterior portion of the neural arch of C-1 in an 8-year-old boy.

FIG 3–29.—Incomplete formation of the neural arch of C-1, seen best in the occipital view (**A**).

FIG 3–30.—Air in the pinna (←) simulating a fracture of the neural arch of C-1 (⇐).

FIG 3–31.—Unilateral absence of a portion of the neural arch of C-1. **A,** defect seen in lateral projection. **B,** defect seen in oblique projection. **C,** normal side for comparison. (Ref: Karasick S, Karasick D, Wechsler RJ: Unilateral spondylolysis of the cervical spine. *Skeletal Radiol* 1983; 9:259.)

FIG 3–32.—Unilateral spondylolysis of C-1 with sclerosis at the site of the lysis, best seen in the center figure (←).

FIG 3–33.—An appearance similar to that in Figure 3–32 may be produced by faulty positioning. **A,** apparent defects in neural arch of C-1 in off-lateral projection. **B,** defects now seen in true lateral projection. **C,** CT shows the neural arch to be intact.

FIG 3–34.—Spondylolysis of C-1 seen in off-lateral projection **(A),** but not in true lateral projection **(B).**

FIG 3–35.—The arcuate foramina formed by calcification of the oblique atlanto-occipital ligaments. The vertebral arteries pass through these foramina. **A,** complete foramen. **B,** incomplete foramen. **C** and **D,** calcification in the oblique atlanto-occipital ligaments, forming incomplete arcuate foramina.

FIG 3–36.—The posterior arches of C-1 (→) and C-2 (↠) seen in the steep Towne projection.

FIG 3–37.—Normal exaggerated density of the posterior elements of C-1 in 7-year-old girl *(left)* and 15-year-old girl *(right)*.

FIG 3–38.—Uptilted neural arch of C-1.

FIG 3–39.—Absence of ossification in the anterior arch of C-1 in a neonate. This is the normal situation in many neonates. (Ref: Dedick AP, Caffey J: Roentgen findings in the skull and chest in 1,030 newborn infants. *Radiology* 1953; 61:13.)

FIG 3–40.—*Left*, apparent absence of the anterior arch of C-1 in a 29-month-old child. Ordinarily this should be evident by 12 months of age. *Right*, CT shows a small ossific nucleus for the anterior arch.

FIG 3–41.—Normal position of the anterior process of C-1 (→) with relationship to the odontoid (↦) when head is in extension. This may be mistaken for a posttraumatic event.

FIG 3–42.—High position of the anterior arch of C-1 may be seen in normal individuals, even with the head in neutral position.

FIG 3–43.—A, double contours of the anterior aspects of C-1 and C-2 due to rotation. B, normal appearance with proper positioning.

FIG 3–44.—Unusual development of C-2 with ossicle arising from neural arch.

FIG 3–45.—Osseous density representing the lateral mass of C-2 thrown into relief by rotation and tilting of the head.

FIG 3–46.—The dens–C-1 interval normally increases with the head in flexion, particularly in children. **A,** flexion. **B,** neutral position. (Ref: Locke GR, Gardner JI, Van Epps EF: Atlas-dens interval in children. *AJR* 1966; 97:135.) The "V" shaped predens space is a normal variation and does not necessarily indicate damage to the transverse ligament. (Ref: Bohrer SP, Klein A, Martin W III: "V" shaped predens space. *Skeletal Radiol* 1985; 14:111.)

FIG 3–47.—The dens–C-1 interval may change in flexion and extension as in this 10-year-old boy. This interval tends to remain fixed in adults. Note the shift of the posterior laminar line as well. (Ref: Swischuk LE: The cervical spine in childhood. *Curr Probl Diagn Radiol* 1987; 13:98.)

FIG 3–48.—Accessory ossicle posterior to C-1 articulating with the neural arch of C-1.

FIG 3–49.—Osseous processes above and below the posterior arch of C-1.

FIG 3–50.—Accessory ossicles above the anterior process of C-1. (Ref: Lombardi G: The occipital vertebra. *AJR* 1961; 86:260).

FIG 3–51.—**A,** simulated ossicle at tip of the odontoid produced by the mastoid tip. **B,** ossicle not seen in AP projection.

FIG 3–52.—Examples of calcification of the anterior longitudinal ligament above the anterior process of C-1.

FIG 3–53.—Calcification of the anterior longitudinal ligament above and below the anterior process of C-1. *Left,* 14-year-old boy; *right,* 44-year-old man.

FIG 3–54.—Five examples of the variable appearance of the accessory ossicle of the anterior arch of the atlas. The laminagram in **B** indicates an articulation with the inferior aspect of the anterior arch of C-1. This articulation may be confused with a fracture. The ossicle should not be confused with calcific tendinitis of the longus colli muscle. (Ref: Haun C: Retropharyngeal tendinitis. *AJR* 1978; 130:1137.) (From Keats TE: Inferior accessory ossicle of the anterior arch of the atlas. *AJR* 1967; 101:834. Used with permission.)

FIG 3–55.—*Left,* the ear lobe simulating calcific tendinitis of the longus colli muscle. *Right,* the ear lobes identified with metallic markers to confirm the nature of the shadow seen in the *left* figure.

FIG 3–56.—Probable calcification in anterior longitudinal ligament below anterior arch of C-1. Compare with Figure 3–52.

FIG 3–57.—Normal variations in the appearance of the lateral masses of C-1. **A,** spur-like configurations of the medial borders. **B,** foramen-like configuration of the medial borders. **C,** pseudofracture. These variants should not be mistaken for manifestations of trauma. (Ref: Meghrouni V, Jacobson G: The pseudonotch of the atlas. *Radiology* 1959; 72:260.)

FIG 3–58.—The pseudonotch of the atlas mistaken for a fracture. These notches form the attachment site of the transverse ligament.

FIG 3–59.—Two examples of developmental bilateral offsets of the lateral masses of C-1 and C-2 in children. This appearance in an adult would be presumptive evidence of fracture of the neural arch of C-1. This entity is believed to be secondary to a disparity of growth of the atlas and axis vertebrae in children and is most commonly seen in children about the age of 4 years. (Ref: Suss RA, Zimmerman RD, Leeds NE: Pseudospread of the atlas: False sign of Jefferson fracture in children. *AJR* 1983; 140:1079.)

FIG 3–60.—The developmental bilateral offset of the lateral masses of C-1 on C-2 may persist in older children as well, as seen in this 6-year-old.

FIG 3–61.—The midline cleft in the odontoid is usually closed at birth. It has persisted in this 4-year-old boy. (Ref: Ogden JA: Radiology of postnatal skeletal development. XII. 2nd cervical vertebra. *Skeletal Radiol* 1984; 12:169).

FIG 3–62.—Normal ossification centers for the tip of the odontoid process. This center appears at age 2 and fuses at 12 years of age. **A,** 5-year-old boy; **B,** 7-year-old boy. Minor variations in width of the interval between the odontoid and the lateral masses, as shown in **B,** due to rotation of the head at the time of filming, should not be mistaken for evidence of trauma (⊣⊢). (Ref: Wortzman G, DeWar FP: Rotary fixation of the atlantoaxial joint: Rotational atlantoaxial subluxation. *Radiology* 1968; 90:479.)

FIG 3–63.—The ossification of the tip of the odontoid (os terminale) in frontal and lateral projections in a 9-year-old boy.

FIG 3–64.—Mach effect produced by the shadow of the tongue, simulating a united ossification center of the tip of the odontoid process.

FIG 3–65.—The synchondrosis of the base of the odontoid process.

FIG 3–66.—The synchondrosis at the base of the odontoid may be mistaken for a fracture in children. The junction usually closes by age 7. **A,** 2-year-old child. **B,** 3-year-old child.

FIG 3–67.—Persistence of a portion of the odontoid synchondrosis in a 13-year-old boy.

FIG 3–68.—Residuals of the odontoid synchrondrosis in a 23-year-old woman.

FIG 3–69.—Residuals of the odontoid synchondroses in a 28-year-old woman.

FIG 3–70.—Sclerosis of the odontoid synchondrosis and asymmetry of the odontoid process.

FIG 3–71.—Fusion of the anterior arch of C-1 to the odontoid in a 3-year-old boy. **A,** plain film. **B,** tomogram. (Ref: Olbrantz K, Bohrer SP: Fusion of the anterior arch of the atlas to dens. *Skeletal Radiol* 1984; 12:21.)

FIG 3–72.—Normal developmental clefts at the base of the odontoid, remnants of the synchondrosis.

FIG 3–73.—Congenital absence of the odontoid process and posterior arch of C-1 detected as an incidental finding. Note characteristic overdevelopment of the anterior arch of C-1, seen in congenital absence of the odontoid and in failure of union of the odontoid.

FIG 3–74.—Failure of union of the odontoid with a separate os odontoideum (→). Note also failure of segmentation of C-2. Os odontoideum is often difficult to differentiate from old odontoid fracture. It is potentially dangerous if excessive motion is present. (Refs: Roback DL: Topics in radiology. *JAMA* 1981; 245:963; and Dawson LG, Smith L: Atlantoaxial subluxation in children due to vertebral anomalies. *J Bone Joint Surg* 1979; 61A:582.)

FIG 3–75.—Two additional examples (two views each) of os odontoideum. Note overgrowth of the anterior arch of C-1. The hypertrophy of the anterior arch is a useful sign in differentiating os odontoideum from acute dens fracture. (Ref: Holt RG, et al: Hypertrophy of C1 anterior arch: Useful sign to distinguish os odontoideum from acute dens fracture. *Radiology* 1989; 173:207.)

FIG 3–76.—*Left*, simulated os odontoideum produced by the lateral masses of C-1. *Center*, tomogram shows the lateral mass that produces the apparent discontinuity of the odontoid. *Right*, tomogram shows no os odontoideum.

FIG 3–77.—Odontoid hypoplasia (←) with large occipital condyles (↔). (Ref: McManners T: Odontoid hypoplasia. *Br J Radiol* 1983; 56:907.)

FIG 3–78.—Odontoid hypoplasia. This entity may be associated with C1–2 instability.

FIG 3–79.—Two examples of anomalous development of the base of the odontoid. Note the corresponding deformity of the lateral masses of C-1.

FIG 3–80.—Asymmetric development of the cerebral condyles and the lateral masses of C-2 as well as the odontoid process. There is also incomplete segmentation of C-2 and C-3.

FIG 3–81.—Asymmetry of development of the lateral masses of C-2 with lateral deviation of the odontoid.

FIG 3–82.—Asymmetry of the lateral masses of C-1 and C-2.

FIG 3–83.—Unusual pointed anterior aspect of the odontoid process, not to be confused with the product of bony erosion (←). **A,** plain film. **B,** laminagram. Note also spur-like extension from superior aspect of the anterior arch of C-1 (�ǂ).

FIG 3–84.—Unusual configuration of the tip of the odontoid process (←). Note also the normal asymmetry of the Luschka joints due to positioning of the head (⇔).

FIG 3–85.—Turbinal configuration of tip of the odontoid process.

FIG 3-86.—Marked "waist" in midodontoid.

FIG 3-87.—Four examples of posterior inclination of the odontoid that should not be confused with fracture. Note characteristic high position of the anterior arch of C-1. (Ref: Swischuk LE, et al: The posterior tilted dens: Normal variation simulating fracture. *Pediatr Radiol* 1979; 8:27.)

FIG 3-88.—Two examples of ossicles about the tip of the odontoid process.

FIG 3-89.—Large ossicle at tip of odontoid process.

FIG 3–90.—A, normal asymmetry of the intervals between the odontoid and the lateral masses of C-1, produced by rotation of the head. **B,** same patient with head in neutral position.

FIG 3–91.—*Left,* the effect of head tilting to the right. The atlas has glided to the patient's right side. The space between the left lateral mass and the dens has decreased, while that on the right has widened. The lateral margins of the lateral atlantoaxial joint spaces are asymmetrical *(arrows).* The spinous processes are deviated to the left. *Right,* CT shows the corresponding asymmetry of the spaces between the lateral masses of C-1 and the dens. (Ref: Harris JH, Edeiken-Monroe B: *The Radiology of Acute Cervical Spine Trauma,* ed 2. Baltimore, Williams & Wilkins, 1987, p 19.)

FIG 3–92.—Altered relationships between the lateral masses of C-1 and the odontoid process resulting from combined rotation and tilting of the head.

FIG 3–93.—Rotation of the head producing unusual elongated appearance of the lateral mass of C-2 *(arrow)*.

FIG 3–94.—Pseudofractures of the odontoid, produced by overlapping shadows of the central maxillary incisors.

FIG 3–95.—Two examples of the lucency between the maxillary and central incisors superimposed on the odontoid process, simulating a split odontoid.

FIG 3–96.—Simulated cleft in the odontoid process produced by midline closure defect in the anterior arch of the atlas.

FIG 3–97.—Closure defect in the anterior arch of C-1 producing apparent fracture of the odontoid process. **A,** open mouth view of the odontoid. **B,** CT scan. (Ref: Chalmers AG: Spondyloschisis of the anterior arch of the atlas. *Br J Radiol* 1985; 58:761.)

FIG 3–98.—Pseudofracture of the body of C-2, produced by overlapping shadows of the teeth.

FIG 3–99.—Pseudofractures of the base of the odontoid, produced by the Mach effect from overlapping shadows of the posterior arch of C-1, the tongue, or the occiput. Each was proved a pseudofracture by laminagraphy. (Ref: Daffner RH: Pseudofracture of the dens: Mach bands. *AJR* 1977; 128:607.)

FIG 3–100.—Pseudofracture of the odontoid, produced by overlapping of base of skull.

FIG 3–101.—Pseudofracture of the odontoid, produced by a vascular groove in the skull.

FIG 3–102.—A, pseudofractures of the transverse processes of C-1 and C-2, produced by Mach bands, probably overlapping the shadow of the anterior tonsillar pillar. B, laminagraphy shows no evidence of fracture.

FIG 3–103.—A, Mach effect from shadows of the lips producing a simulated fracture. B, reexamination shows no evidence of fracture.

FIG 3–104.—Remnants of the synchondroses of the primary ossification centers of C-2 (→). Note also the pseudofracture of the base of the odontoid (↦).

FIG 3–105.—Pseudofracture of the body of C-2, produced by overlapping pharyngeal soft tissue shadows.

FIG 3–106.—Persistent apophysis for the transverse process of C-2. (Ref: Kohler A, Zimmer EA: *Borderlands of the Normal and Early Pathologic in Skeletal Roentgenology,* ed 3. New York, Grune & Stratton, 1968, p 311.)

FIG 3–107.—The C-2 "target" composite shadow is a projectional variant formed by a composite image related to the facets. (Ref: Nicolet V, et al: C2 "target": Composite shadow. *AJNR* 1984; 5:331.) Disruption of this ring shadow is a good indicator of a low (type III) odontoid fracture. (Ref: Harris JH, et al: Low (type III) odontoid fracture: A new radiographic sign. *Radiology* 1984; 153:353.)

FIG 3–108.—In the younger patient, the C-2 target shadow may appear as several rings, as shown in this 13-year-old boy.

FIG 3–109.—Spina bifida of C-2 simulating fracture.

FIG 3–110.—Pseudofracture of C-2 produced by overlapping of large uncinate processes. (Ref: Daffner R: Pseudofracture of the cervical vertebral body. *Skeletal Radiol* 1986; 15:295.)

FIG 3–111.—Very large uncovertebral processes in a 33-year-old woman.

FIG 3–112.—Normal contour alterations in the neural arch of C-2 may produce pseudofractures.

FIG 3–113.—The superimposed lobe of the ear may produce shadows similar to those shown in Figure 3–112 and may simulate fracture (→). Note in **B** the cleft in the anterior aspect of the vertebral body, which is probably a remnant of the synchondrosis for the odontoid process (↠).

FIG 3–114.—*Left,* many patients exhibit a shallow groove at the superior aspect of the neural arch of C-2 (←) that could be mistaken for a hangman's fracture. *Right,* in flexion these grooves are seen bilaterally. The physiologic subluxation of C-2 on C-3 reinforces the impression of a hangman's fracture.

FIG 3–115.—An additional example of the groove of the neural arch of C-2 that can be mistaken for fracture.

FIG 3–116.—*Left,* simulated fracture of the neural arch of C-2 produced by rotation. *Right,* CT shows no fracture.

FIG 3–117.—Simulated fracture of C-2, produced by slight rotation with superimposition of the superior articular process on the vertebral body.

FIG 3–118.—A, simulated fracture produced by Mach effect of the odontoid. **B,** tomogram shows no fracture of C-1. Note pseudofracture of C-2) (↔).

FIG 3–119.—In some patients, the C-2 vertebra is larger in its inferior portions than the adjacent C-3 vertebra, giving a pseudo "fat C-2 sign" that indicates a vertical C-2 body fracture. (Refs: Bohrer SP: Pseudosigns in cervical spine trauma radiology. *Contemp Diagn Radiol* 1989, vol 12, no. 13; and Smoker WRK, Dolan KD: The "fat C2": A sign of fracture. *AJR* 1987; 148:609).

FIG 3–120.—Anomalous articulation between C-2 and C-3.

FIG 3–121.—A, simulated fusion of posterior elements of C-2 and C-3 produced by rotation. **B,** repeat film shows no abnormality at C2–3, but apparent fusion now appears at C-5 and C-6.

FIG 3–122.—The foramen transversarium. The central density is a portion of the vertebra projected through the lucency of the foramen.

FIG 3–123.—Developmental cleft in anterior aspect of C-2.

FIG 3–124.—Three examples of incomplete segmentation of C2–3, commonly called congenital block vertebra. Occasionally, this may predispose to early degenerative spondylosis at the next lower intervertebral disc. (Ref: de Graaff R: Congenital block vertebrae C2-C3 in patients with cervical myelopathy. *Acta Neurochir* 1982; 61:111.)

FIG 3–125.—Failure of segmentation of the neural arches of C-2 and C-3.

FIG 3–126.—Incomplete segmentation of C2–3 with a huge irregular foramen between the neural arches.

FIG 3–127.—Partial segmentation of C2–3, originally diagnosed as a fracture.

FIG 3–128.—Block vertebrae are often associated with defects in architecture. Note the failure of fusion of the lateral mass of C-2 in the AP film **(B).** Rarely this anomaly may be associated with radiculopathy. (Ref: Okada K, et al: Cervical radiculopathy associated with an anomaly of the cervical vertebrae. *J Bone Joint Surg* 1988; 70A:1399.)

FIG 3–129.—Nonsegmentation of C-3 and C-4 with asymmetric development of the pedicles.

FIG 3–130.—Partial segmentation of C2–3 **(A)** with spina bifida **(B)** seen in a 9-year-old child.

FIG 3–131.—*Left,* partial nonsegmentation of C-6 and C-7 mistaken for acquired narrowing of the intervertebral disc in a 35-year-old man. C-2 and C-3 are also nonsegmented. *Right,* the spina bifida occulta of these two vertebrae indicates the developmental nature of the finding at C-6 and C-7 (arrow).

FIG 3–132.—**A,** unilateral closure defect in the lamina on the left side of C-2. **B,** opposite side for comparison.

FIG 3–133.—Anomalous ossicle between the spinous processes of C-2 and C-3. *Left*, plain film. *Right*, tomogram.

FIG 3–134.— Pseudosubluxation of C-2 on C-3 in a 6-year-old boy (A). This is the normal area of maximum movement in the child and pseudosubluxation is regularly seen in flexion. View with the head in neutral position (B) shows normal relationships. (Ref: Jacobson G, Beeckler HH: Pseudosubluxation of the axis in children. *AJR* 1959; 82:472.)

FIG 3–135.—Another example of pseudosubluxation of C-2 on C-3 in a 4-year-old boy. Note neck in flexion. The posterior cervical line is useful in differentiating true subluxation from pseudosubluxation of C-2 on C-3 (see Fig 3–160). (Ref: Swischuk LE: Anterior displacement of C2 in children. Physiologic or pathologic. *Radiology* 1977; 122:759.)

FIG 3–136.—Physiologic subluxation of C-2 on C-3 may also occur in adults. **A,** 20-year-old man. **B,** 34-year-old woman. (Ref: Harrison RB, et al: Pseudosubluxation of the axis in young adults. *J Can Assoc Radiol* 1980; 31:176.)

FIG 3–137.—Physiologic subluxation may occasionally be seen in cervical extension as well as in flexion, as in this 20-year-old man. **A,** neutral position. **B,** flexion. **C,** extension. (Ref: Harris JH: Radiographically subtle soft tissue injuries of the cervical spine. *Curr Probl Diagn Radiol* 1989; 18:166).

FIG 3–138.—Normal variations in curvature of the cervical spine, depending on head position in the same patient on the same day. Such variations should not necessarily be taken as evidence of posttraumatic muscle spasm.

FIG 3–139.—Normal cervical spine. **A,** neutral position. **B,** flexion. Note the striking alteration in curvature that can be produced with only slight alteration in head position.

FIG 3–140.—Physiologic subluxation may occur at multiple levels in flexion, particularly in children. **A,** note anterior subluxation of C-2 on C-3, C-3 on C-4, and C-4 on C-5 in a child. Posterior cervical line is intact. **B,** normal alignment in neutral position. (Ref: Swischuk LE: The cervical spine in childhood. *Curr Probl Diagn Radiol* 1984; 13:10.)

FIG 3–141.—*Left,* multiple physiologic subluxations on flexion in 9-year-old boy. *Center,* neutral position. *Right,* extension.

FIG 3–142.—Physiologic subluxation of C-2 on C-3 and C-3 on C-4 in a 17-year-old boy on flexion.

FIG 3–143.—**A** and **B**, physiologic anterior "slipping" of cervical vertebrae on flexion (**A**) and correction on extension (**B**). **C** and **D**, physiologic posterior "slipping" of cervical vertebrae on extension (**C**) and correction on flexion (**D**). These minor degrees of "malalignment" with extremes of motion are not necessarily abnormal in themselves, particularly if the "slipping" occurs at multiple levels in continuity. (Ref: Scher AT: Anterior subluxation: An unstable position. *AJR* 1979; 133:275.)

FIG 3–144.—Spondylolysis of the neural arch of C-4 simulating fracture. **A,** plain film, lateral. **B,** tomogram. **C,** CT scan. (Ref: Forsberg DA: Cervical spondylolysis. *AJR* 1990; 154:751).

FIG 3–145.—**A,** an example of the simulated fracture of the posterior neural arch of C-2, produced by rotation. **B,** corrected position. No fracture is seen.

FIG 3–146.—A, simulated fracture of the posterior neural arch of C-3 produced by rotation. B, corrected position. No fracture is seen.

FIG 3–147.—A, simulated fracture of the neural arch of C-3, produced by rotation. B, repeat examination with correction of rotation shows restitution to normal appearance. Note also the absence of lordotic curve in A. This is a common variation, especially between the ages of 8 and 16 years. (Ref: Cattell HS, Filtzer DL: Pseudosubluxation and other normal variations in the cervical spine in children. *J Bone Joint Surg* 1965; 47A:1295.)

FIG 3–148.—A, pseudofracture of the neural arch of the type shown in Figure 3–147 (→). B, repeat film shows disappearance of the pseudofracture shown in A and the appearance of the pseudofracture shown in Figure 3–149 (↠).

FIG 3–149.—*Left,* pseudofracture of the inferior articulating process of C-3. *Right,* true lateral shows that the pseudofracture is due to the overlapping shadows of the inferior articulating processes.

FIG 3–150.—Simulated fracture of C-3 due to rotation.

FIG 3–151.—Simulated rotary dislocation of C-3 resulting from positioning. Note that the facets are in proper relationship above and below.

FIG 3–152.—Two examples of the pseudovacuum of the cervical intervertebral disc related to the Mach band phenomenon. This should not be confused with a true vacuum sign of an intervertebral disc injury. (Ref: Daffner RH, Gehweiler JA: Pseudovacuum of the cervical intervertebral disc. *AJR* 1981; 137:737. Used by permission.)

FIG 3–153.—Wide spacing between spinous processes of C-3 and C-4, which might be misconstrued as evidence of flaring due to soft tissue injury. Note lack of change between flexion (**A**) and neutral position (**B**). This pseudofanning occurs most commonly at C3–4. (Ref: Bohrer SP: Pseudosigns in cervical spine trauma radiology. *Contemp Diagn Radiol* 1989; vol 12, no. 13.

FIG 3–154.—Absence of the posterior elements of C-2.

FIG 3–155.—Absence of portions of the posterior arch of C-4.

FIG 3–156.—Uptilted spinous process of C-5 might be misconstrued as evidence of soft tissue injury between C-6 and C-7.

FIG 3–157.—Upturned spinous process originally interpreted as evidence of ligamentous injury with flaring of the spinous processes.

FIG 3–158.—Normal wedge shape of juvenile cervical vertebral bodies, which should not be confused with compression fracture.

FIG 3–159.—Wedge-shaped vertebral bodies in a 13-year-old boy. Note particularly the marked wedging of C-3, mistaken for a compression fracture.

FIG 3–160.—Normal retention of wedged configuration of C-3 in a 54-year-old woman. Note also that the base of the spinous process of C-2 (→) lies slightly posterior to that of C-1 and C-3 (⊣⊢). This is a normal variation that may be seen in children as well and should not be mistaken for evidence of subluxation. (Ref: Kattan KR: Backward "displacement" of the spinolaminal line at C-2: A normal variation. *AJR* 1977; 129:289.)

FIG 3–161.—Backward "displacement" of the spinolaminal line at C-2 is a normal variation in both children and adults and should not be mistaken for evidence of subluxation. (Ref: Kattan K: Backward "displacement" of the spinolaminal line at C-2: A normal variation. *AJR* 1977; 129:289).

FIG 3–162.—Normal retention of wedged configuration of C-3, C-4, and C-5 in an adult.

FIG 3–163.—Unusual configuration of C-3. Tomography showed no evidence of fracture.

FIG 3–164.—Normal wedged appearance of C-5 in a 33-year-old man that should not be mistaken for a compression fracture. Note absence of condensation of bone or buckling of the anterior cortex. (Refs: Kattan K, Pais MJ: Some borderlands of the cervical spine. *Skeletal Radiol* 1982; 8:1; and Kim KS, et al: Pitfalls in plain film diagnosis of cervical spine injuries: False positive interpretation. *Surg Neurol* 1986; 25:381.)

FIG 3–165.—Four additional examples of unusual configurations of C-5 that might be misconstrued as evidence of trauma.

FIG 3–166.—Simulated destructive lesion of the third and fourth cervical vertebrae, produced by slight rotation at the time of filming.

FIG 3–167.—The normal secondary ossification centers of the vertebrae in a 14-year-old boy.

FIG 3–168.—Closing secondary ossification centers in a 16-year-old boy.

FIG 3–169.—Anterior and posterior ring apophyses of the vertebrae. (Ref: Anni G, Hudson JM: Posterior ring apophyses of the cervical spine. *AJR* 1982; 139:383.)

FIG 3–170.—Unfused uncinate apophysis, which might be mistaken for fracture. (Ref: Shaff RE, et al: Lateral hyperflexion injuries of the cervical spine. *Skeletal Radiol* 1978; 3:73.)

FIG 3–171.—Three examples of cervical limbus vertebrae. When these elements appear in adult life they probably represent calcification in the anulus fibrosus secondary to stress. (Ref: Kerns S, et al: Annulus fibrosus calcification in the cervical spine: Radiologic-pathologic correlation. *Skeletel Radiol* 1986; 15:605.)

FIG 3–172.—Ununited ossification centers at the inferior articular process of C-4 *(left and center).* Ununited ossification centers of the fifth and sixth cervical vertebrae, which simulate fracture (limbus vertebrae) *(right).*

FIG 3–173.—Ununited ossification center of the inferior articular process of C-5.

FIG 3–174.—Ununited ossification center of the inferior articular process of C-6.

FIG 3–175.—Ununited ossification centers of transverse processes of last two cervical vertebrae in a 38-year-old man.

FIG 3–176.—Fissure in the spinous process of C-2, simulating a fracture. The *upper arrow* indicates the arcuate foramen.

FIG 3–177.—Accessory ossification centers at the tip of the spinous process of C-3. **A,** lateral projection. **B,** oblique projection.

FIG 3–178.—A bifid spinous process (→) may project into the neural foramen and simulate a fracture (⇢).

FIG 3–179.—An example of the confusing appearance of the neural foramina (→), produced by bifid spinous processes (⇢).

FIG 3–180.—A spinous process bifid in the horizontal plane.

FIG 3–181.—A, facet seen in the oblique projection and mistaken for fracture of the lamina. B, tomogram shows no fracture. (Ref: Zielinski CJ, Griffith JL: A joint shadow in the cervical spine presenting as a vertebral body fracture. *Spine* 1987; 12:595.)

FIG 3–182.—A facet seen in the oblique projection resembling a fracture.

FIG 3–183.—A, simulated fractures, of laminae of C-5 produced by facets. **B,** tomogram shows no fracture.

FIG 3–184.—Congenital absence of the pedicle of C-5 on the right. Compare oblique projection **(B)** with normal side **(C)** and note the enlarged foramen on the abnormal side (see Fig 3–225). (Ref: Chapman M: Congenital absence of cervical pedicle. *Skeletal Radiol* 1976; 1:65.)

FIG 3–185.—Congenital absence of the pedicle on the left at C-5 *(arrows)*. A spina bifida occulta is also present **(A–C)**. Compare oblique projection **(C)** with normal side **(D)**. **E,** CT scan shows absence of pedicle and spina bifida occulta. **F,** CT scan shows the facets to be in opposite planes. This can be seen in **A** as well. (Ref: Wiener MD, et al: Congenital absence of a cervical spine pedicle: Clinical and radiologic findings. *AJR* 1990; 155:1037.)

FIG 3–186.— Absent pedicle at C-6 on the left. **A,** AP. **B** and **C,** oblique. **D,** CT. **E,** PA myelogram shows conjoined root sleeves *(arrow)* (see Fig 3–353).

FIG 3–187.—Anomalous articulation between transverse processes of C-5 and C-6 due to elongation of the anterior tubercle. (Ref: Applebaum Y, et al: Elongation of the anterior tubercle of a cervical vertebral transverse process: An unusual variant. *Skeletal Radiol* 1983; 10:265.)

FIG 3–188.—A similar anomalous articulation between the transverse processes of C-5 and C-6 can be seen with incomplete segmentation of these two vertebral bodies.

FIG 3–189.—Anomalous articulation between the transverse processes of C-5 and C-6 similar to that of Figure 3–188 with CT confirmation *(arrows)*.

FIG 3–190.—Three examples of the variability of vertebral body size in a given individual.

FIG 3–191.—Sclerosis of the pedicles and posterolateral aspects of the vertebral bodies in a 36-year-old woman, best seen in the oblique projection. This is apparently not related to degenerative spondylosis.

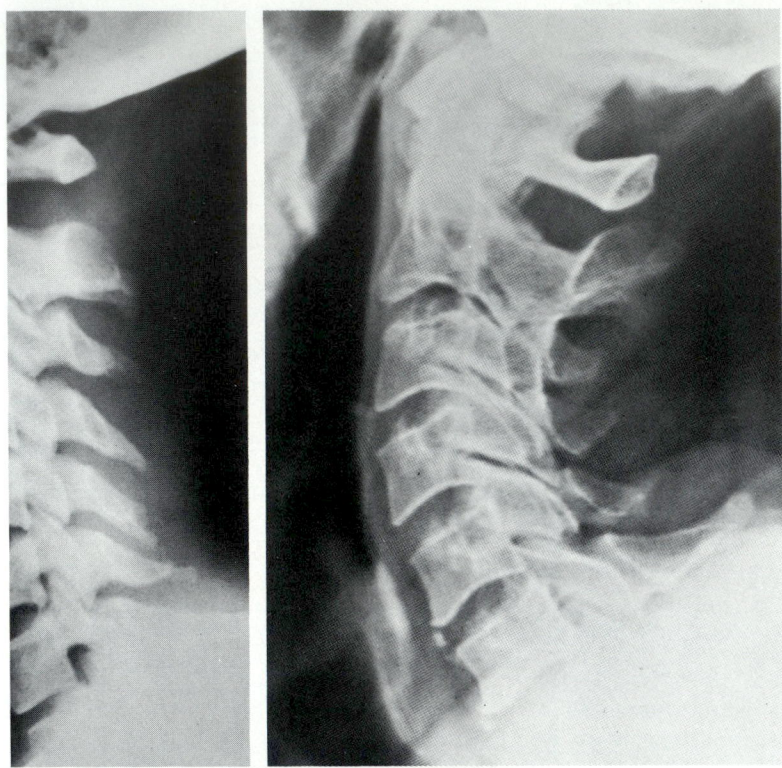

FIG 3–192.— Three examples of the normal variability of size and configuration of spinous processes.

FIG 3–193.—Bifid spinous processes of C-5 and C-6, which may be mistaken for fracture.

FIG 3–194.—Ossicle between C-5 and C-6, probably ligamentous.

FIG 3–195.—Calcification of the posterior longitudinal ligament. This may or may not be of significance. (Ref: Minagi H, Gronner AT: Calcification of the posterior longitudinal ligament: A cause of cervical myelopathy. *AJR* 1969; 105;365.)

FIG 3–196.—**A,** simulated calcification of the posterior spinal ligament produced by rotation. **B,** not seen with correct positioning.

FIG 3–197.—Calcification of the ligamentum nuchae at the base of the skull.

FIG 3–198.—Calcification of the ligamentum nuchae.

FIG 3–199.—Two examples of simulated fusion of the apophyseal joints, produced by projection.

FIG 3–200.—Failure of union of the apophysis of the tip of the spinous process of C-7 simulating a fracture.

FIG 3–201.—Ununited apophysis of the spinous process of C-6 with an anomalous articulation.

FIG 3–202.—Three examples of normal elongation of the transverse process of C-5 and C-6, producing an unusual appearance anterior to the vertebral bodies (see Fig 3–187). (Ref: Laypayowker MS: An unusual variant of the cervical spine. *AJR* 1960; 83:656.)

FIG 3–203.—Oblique projection of the cervical spine showing the anterior tubercle of the transverse process, the structure responsible for the shadows in Figure 3–202.

FIG 3–204.—Large transverse processes with attempts to form ribs at C-5 and C-7.

FIG 3–205.—*Left,* long transverse process of C-6 simulating a fracture *(arrow)*. *Right,* oblique projection shows the elongated transverse process *(arrow)*.

FIG 3–206.—*Left*, ring-like shadow produced by lateral elements of the vertebra with slight rotation at the time of filming. *Right*, true lateral projection does not show the ring shadow.

FIG 3–207.—Simulated fractures of vertebral bodies produced by the shadows of the transverse processes.

FIG 3–208.—Block vertebrae at C5-6 with spina bifida.

FIG 3–209.—Nonsegmented vertebrae at C3-4 and C5-6. Oblique projection shows resulting deformity of intervertebral foramina.

FIG 3–211.—Failure of segmentation of C5-6.

FIG 3–210.—Partial segmentation error at C4-5. Note underdevelopment of the vertebral bodies.

FIG 3–212.—Block vertebrae of C6-7 with marked elongation of the spinous processes.

FIG 3–213.—Posterior tilt of the spinolaminal line of C-6, which should not be confused with the effect of an intraspinal lesion.

FIG 3–214.—Two examples of developmental spur-like processes arising from the posterior portion of the neural arches of C-5 and C-6.

FIG 3–215.—Two examples of normal notching of the apophyseal joint surfaces of the lower cervical spine, not to be mistaken for erosion or fracture. (Ref: Keats TE, Johnstone WH: Notching of the lamina of C-7: A proposed mechanism. *Skeletal Radiol* 1982; 7:273.)

FIG 3–216.—*Left,* the laminar notch at C-7. *Right,* in extension, note how the inferior articular process fits into the notch.

FIG 3–217.—*Left,* the laminar notch at C-7 mistaken for a fracture. *Right,* tomogram shows no fracture.

FIG 3–218.—Notches in the superior extremity of the superior articulating processes of C-6 and C-7, presumably developmental, detected as an incidental finding. **A,** plain film. **B,** tomogram.

FIG 3–219.—Simulated fracture of C-5 produced by uncovertebral joint degeneration. (Ref: Goldberg RP, et al: The cervical split: A pseudofracture. *Skeletal Radiol* 1982; 7:267.)

FIG 3–220.—Multiple pseudofractures due to uncovertebral degeneration.

FIG 3–221.—Air in the pyriform sinuses simulating destructive lesions of the cervical spine.

FIG 3–222.—Three examples of simulated destructive lesions of the lower cervical spine, produced by projection.

FIG 3–223.—Spina bifida of C-7 simulating a fracture. **A,** plain film. **B,** tomogram.

FIG 3–224.—Spina bifida of C-7 with double spinous processes.

FIG 3–225.—Congenital absence of the C-7 pedicle on the right (←). A spina bifida occulta is also present (↔) (**A–C**). Compare oblique projection (**C**) with normal side (**D**). This congenital lesion may be mistaken for an acquired one (see Fig 3–184). (Refs: Chapman M: Congenital absence of cervical pedicle. *Skeletal Radiol* 1976; 1:65; and Van Dijk Azn R, et al: The absent cervical pedicle syndrome. *Neuroradiology* 1987; 29:69.)

FIG 3–226.—The omovertebral bone between C-5 and T-1 unassociated with Sprengel's deformity.

FIG 3–227.—*Top left*, the lateral elements of C-6 projected slightly caudad show two apophyseal joints that were misinterpreted as fractures. *Top right and bottom*, oblique projections show no abnormality.

FIG 3–228.—The normal "bone in bone" appearance of the thoracic vertebrae in a neonate.

FIG 3–229.—Normal thoracic spine at 1 month of age. The "bone in bone" appearance is present, and the large central notches on the anterior surface of the vertebrae are normal at this age.

FIG 3–230.—Normal neonatal thoracic spine, showing "sandwich" appearance due to large venous sinuses.

FIG 3–231.—The dense end-plates of the vertebral bodies produce an unusual appearance in the frontal film of a 4-month-old child.

FIG 3–232.—Prominent residual venous sinus "holes" in older child's thoracic spine.

FIG 3–233.—Normal thoracic spine in a 5-year-old child. The vascular stripes in the center of the anterior portion of the vertebral body and the notches in the anterior corners of the vertebrae are normal at this age.

FIG 3–234.—The appearance of the venous grooves in the frontal projection of a newborn.

FIG 3–235.—Four examples of residual venous sinus grooves in adults.

FIG 3–236.—*Left*, residual venous sinus grooves may add to the impression of a compression fracture in a poorly positioned lateral projection. Better lateral projection *(right)* shows no fracture.

FIG 3–237.—Persistence of the posterior vascular notch in a 33-year-old man.

FIG 3–238.—Normal "step" defects on the anterior surfaces of juvenile vertebrae. **A,** 4 years of age. **B,** 7 years of age.

FIG 3–239.—Ossification centers at the distal ends of the transverse processes of T-1 in an adolescent.

FIG 3–240.—Nonunited ossification centers at the distal ends of the transverse processes of T-1 in an adult.

FIG 3–241.—Two examples of unilateral persistence of the ossification centers of the transverse processes in young adults.

FIG 3–242.—Unfused epiphyses of the transverse processes of T-1 (←) and at the medial ends of the first ribs (⊢) in a 14-year-old boy.

FIG 3–243.—Failure of union of the apophysis for the tip of the spinous process of T-1.

FIG 3–244.—Two examples of how the lateral elements of T-1 produce apparent sclerosis of a portion of the vertebral body and may simulate a metastatic deposit.

FIG 3–245.—Shadow produced by the normal posterior angulation of the transverse process of T-1.

FIG 3–246.—Apparent narrowing of interpedicular distance at the thoracolumbar junction in a 2-week-old infant due to the normal thoracolumbar kyphosis and resultant magnification effect.

FIG 3–247.—Narrow pedicles in a young woman on a developmental basis.

FIG 3–248.—Delicate bone structure in a young woman with thin pedicles, simulating pedicular erosion.

FIG 3–249.—Minor scoliosis, producing simulated pedicle erosion.

FIG 3–250.—Localized scoliosis, simulating pedicle erosion.

FIG 3–251.—Asymmetry of the pedicles of the lower thoracic spine. This is seen as a normal variation in 7% of normal individuals. The measured interpediculate distance does not exceed 2 SD from the mean in this normal variation. (Ref: Benzian SR, et al: Pediculate thinning: A normal variant at the thoracolumbar junction. *Br J Radiol* 1971; 44: 936.)

FIG 3–252.—Pedicle thinning at the thoracolumbar junction may be extreme and may even be associated with concave medial borders. The absence of pertinent clinical findings should suggest this recognized normal variation. (Ref: Charlton OP, et al: Pedicle thinning at the thoracolumbar junction: A normal variant. *AJR* 1980; 134:825.)

FIG 3-253.—Spina bifida occulta of C-7 and T-1 with double spinous processes.

FIG 3-254.—Spina bifida of T-1, simulating a fracture.

FIG 3-255.—Spina bifida of the spinous process of T-12.

FIG 3–257.—Spina bifida occulta of T-11 and T-12 and L-1 and L-2.

FIG 3–256.—Thoracic lordosis, a normal variation, in a 54-year-old man.

FIG 3–258.—*Left*, bulbous spinous process of T-11 simulating a mass. *Right*, detailed view shows identity of the shadow.

FIG 3–259.—Spina bifida of T-11 and T-12.

FIG 3–260.—Spina bifida occulta of T-12.

FIG 3–261.—Limbus vertebra at T-10 in a 24-year-old man.

FIG 3–262.—Two examples of failure of segmentation of the thoracic vertebrae. Partial development of the intervertebral discs is seen. This should not be confused with the effects of inflammatory spondylitis.

FIG 3–263.—Congenital butterfly vertebra. Note overgrowth of adjacent vertebra.

FIG 3–264.—Partial hemivertebra mistaken for a calcified intervertebral disc. Note deformity of adjacent vertebral bodies.

FIG 3–265.—Hemivertebra, originally misinterpreted as a cystic lesion of the vertebra. Note that in the frontal plane, one can see vertebral end-plates only on the patient's right side *(arrows)*.

FIG 3–266.—Another case of hemivertebra with more obvious changes than in Figure 3–265. Note the absence of a pedicle on the patient's left side. (Ref: McMaster MJ, David CV: Hemivertebra as a cause of scoliosis. *J Bone Joint Surg* 1986; 68B:588.)

FIG 3–268.—Pseudofractures of the thoracic spine. **A,** superimposition of the glenoid process of the scapula on the thoracic spine, simulating a vertebral compression fracture. **B,** pseudofracture of the second thoracic vertebra, produced by superimposition of the superior margin of the manubrium.

FIG 3–267.—Asymptomatic calcification of the nucleus pulposus in a young adult. This is generally asymptomatic. When it occurs in the cervical region in children, it may be associated with signs and symptoms, but is self-limited. (Ref: Melnick JC, Silverman FN: Intervertebral disk calcification in childhood. *Radiology* 1963; 80:399.)

FIG 3–269.—Four examples of how the interarticulating facets of the spine may simulate bulging anuli or paraspinous masses (see Fig 3–319).

FIG 3–270.—"Bumpy spine," produced by hypertrophy of the costovertebral articulations.

FIG 3–271.—Nodular densities, produced by the vertebral laminae.

FIG 3–272.—Atypical joint-like union of the transverse processes at the level of T-4 and T-5 (see Fig 3–187).

FIG 3–273.— Anomalous articulation between the transverse processes of T-3 and T-4 (see Figs 3–187 and 3–272).

FIG 3–274.— Anomalous articulation between T-5 and T-6 that can be seen in the lateral projection as well.

FIG 3–275.—*Left,* anomalous articulation between the transverse processes of T-11 and T-12 mistaken for a mediastinal mass. *Right,* spot film shows the anomalous articulation.

FIG 3–276.—Anomalous articulation between the rib and the adjacent transverse process.

FIG 3–277.—Apparent destructive lesion of the rib, produced by superimposition of the spinous process (*arrow*).

FIG 3–278.—Bilateral styloid processes of T-9.

FIG 3–279.—Developmental notch in the inferior articulating process of T-12 is a common anatomic variant at this level.

FIG 3–281.—*Left*, target pedicle of T-12. This appearance is produced by superimposition of the shadows of the inferior and lateral tubercules on the shadow of the pedicle. *Center*, absent pedicle at T–12. Frontal film shows absence of pedicular ring shadow. *Right*, absent pedicle at T–12. Tomogram shows incomplete shadows of the pedicles as seen above and below. (Refs: Ehara S, et al: Target pedicle of T12: Radiologic-anatomic correlation. *Radiology* 1990; 174:871; Manaster BJ, Norman A: CT diagnosis of thoracic pedicle aplasia. *J Comput Assist Tomogr* 1983; 7:1090; and Lederman RA, Kaufman RA: Complete absence and hypoplasia of pedicles of the thoracic spine. *Skeletal Radiol* 1986; 15:219.)

FIG 3–280.—Thoracic notochordal remnants in a 15-year-old boy (see Fig 3–287).

FIG 3–282.—The costovertebral articulation superimposed on the body of T-12.

FIG 3–283.—Two examples of coronal cleft vertebrae in neonates. These occur more commonly in males and most often in the lumbar region.

FIG 3–284.—The normal "bone in bone" appearance of the neonate.

FIG 3–285.—Normal variation in pedicle size. The interpediculate distance in this variation does not exceed two standard deviations from the mean (see Figs 3–251 and 3–252). (Ref: Benzian SR, et al: Pediculate thinning: A normal variant of the thoracolumbar junction. *Br J Radiol* 1971; 44:936.)

FIG 3–286.—Congenitally wide thoracolumbar spinal canal unassociated with neurologic signs or symptoms. **A** and **B**, plain film—large canal with thin pedicles. **C** and **D**, myelogram—large dural sac. **E** and **F**, CT scans—large spinal canal (see Fig 3–3). (Ref: Patel NP, et al: Radiology of lumbar vertebral pedicles: Variants, anomalies and pathologic conditions. *Radiographics* 1987; 7:101.)

FIG 3–288.—Notochordal remnants producing balloon discs. (Ref: Tsuji H, et al: Developmental balloon discs of the lumbar spine in healthy subjects. *Spine* 1985; 10:907.)

FIG 3–287.—Two examples of end-plate depressions secondary to notochordal remnants. Indentations of this type in the end-plates of normal vertebrae of young people indicate the site of the notochordal recession into the intervertebral disc. They should be differentiated from Schmorl's nodes. **A,** a 27-year-old man. **B,** a 12-year-old girl. (Ref: Dietz GW, Christensen EE: Normal "Cupid's bow" contour of the lower lumbar vertebrae. *Radiology* 1976; 121:577.)

FIG 3–289.—Central radiolucency within the body of L-4 found as an incidental finding, probably representing a notochordal remnant.

FIG 3–291.—Incomplete closure of the neural arches in the lower dorsal and upper lumbar spine.

FIG 3–290.—Unusually tall intervertebral discs in a 31-year-old woman.

FIG 3–292.—Pseudospondylolysis is seen at L-2 and L-3 in perfectly positioned lateral projections, and results from superimposition of the transverse processes. *Left*, pseudospondylolysis at L-2 and L-3 in a true lateral projection. *Center*, the defects disappear when a minor degree of obliquity is present. *Left*, pseudospondylolysis in an infant. (From El-Khoury GY, et al: Pseudospondylolysis. *Radiology* 1981; 139:72. Used by permission.)

FIG 3–293.—Simulated fractures of the transverse processes, produced by the crossing shadow of the psoas muscle.

FIG 3–294.—Absence of the transverse process of the left side of L-1.

FIG 3–295.—Unconnected ribs at L-1 bilaterally.

FIG 3–296.—Bilateral styloid processes of L-1.

FIG 3–297.—Unilateral styloid process of L-1.

FIG 3–298.—Bilateral styloid process of L-4. These accessory processes arise posterior to the base of the superior articular facet. (Ref: Kohler A, Zimmer EA: *Borderlands of the Normal and Early Pathologic in Skeletal Roentgenology,* ed 3. New York, Grune & Stratton, 1968, p 338.)

FIG 3–299.—Unilateral styloid process of L-4 (←). Note normal "Cupid's bow" configuration of inferior plate of L-4 (→), a normal variation. (Ref: Dietz GW, Christensen EE: Normal "Cupid's bow" contour of the lower lumbar vertebrae. *Radiology* 1976; 121:577.)

FIG 3–300.—Ptotic transverse process of L-3. This variant may easily be mistaken for a fracture.

Fig 3–301.—Congenital absence of the transverse process on the left side of L-4.

FIG 3–302.—Anomalous articulation between the transverse processes of L-3 and L-4.

FIG 3–303.—Two examples of pseudarthrosis between the transverse processes of L-3 and L-4. (Ref: Yoslow W, Becker MH: Osseous bridges between the transverse processes of the lumbar spine: Report of three cases and review of the literature. *J Bone Joint Surg* 1968; 50A:513.)

FIG 3–304.—Very large anomalous articulation between the transverse processes of L-3 and L-4. *Left,* AP projection. *Center,* lateral projection. *Right,* oblique projection.

FIG 3–305.—Transverse process of L-3 seen in cross-section.

FIG 3–306.—Cephalad-directed transverse process of L-4.

FIG 3–307.—Failure of union of the transverse process of L-1 with the vertebral body.

FIG 3–308.—Abortive rib formation at L-2.

FIG 3–309.—Lumbar rib. (Courtesy of Dr. Gary M. Guebert.)

FIG 3–310.—Persistence of the apophysis of the transverse process of L-5.

FIG 3–311.—Calcification of the iliolumbar ligaments.

FIG 3–312.—Separate ossification center for transverse process of L-5.

FIG 3–313.—Ununited secondary ossification center of the end of the superior articulating process of L-5.

FIG 3–314.—Persistent apophysis of the mamillary process of L-4.

FIG 3–315.—Ununited ossification center of the end of the inferior articulating process of L-4, which may be mistaken for fracture. **A,** frontal projection. **B,** oblique projection.

FIG 3–316.—Ununited ossification center of the inferior articulating process of L-3.

FIG 3–317.—Bilateral failure of union of the ossification centers of the inferior articulating processes of L-3.

FIG 3–318.—Failure of fusion of the ossification center of the superior articulating process of L-3.

FIG 3–319.—The facets between L-4 and L-5, simulating an osseous or soft tissue mass (see Fig 3–269).

FIG 3–320.— Absence of the inferior articulating process of L-3. (Refs: Arcomano JP, Karas S: Congenital absence of the lumbosacral articular processes. *Skeletal Radiol* 1982; 8:133; and Phillips MR, Keagy RD: Congenital absence of lumbar articular facets with computerized axial tomography documentation. *Spine* 1988; 13:676.)

FIG 3–321.—**A** and **B,** apparent bilateral spondylolysis of L-5 due to projection. **C** and **D,** films made with 15-degree cephalad angulation show no spondylolysis.

FIG 3–322.—**A,** bowel gas simulating spondylolysis of L-2. **B,** repeated examination clarifies the issue.

FIG 3–323.—"Pig snout" pedicle results from superimposition of the shadows of the pedicle and an unusual downward projection of the distal end of the transverse process. (Courtesy of Dr. W.E. Litterer.) (Ref: Patel NP, et al: Radiology of lumbar vertebral pedicles: Variants, anomalies and pathologic conditions. *Radiographics* 1987; 7:101.)

FIG 3–324.—The two-eyed Scotty dog. The second "eye" is created by a prominent mamillary process. (Ref: Resnik CS, et al: The two-eyed Scotty dog: A normal anatomic variant. *Radiology* 1983; 149:680.)

FIG 3–326.—Congenital absence of the left pedicle of L-3. **A,** plain film. **B,** CT scan. (Ref: Wortzman G, Steinhardt MI: Congenitally absent lumbar pedicle: A reappraisal. *Radiology* 1984; 152:713.)

FIG 3–327.—Congenital absence of the pedicle on the right side of L-4 with incomplete segmentation of L-3 and L-4. **A** and **B,** plain films. **C** and **D,** tomograms. Note the huge intervertebral foramen in **D.** (Ref: Mac-Leod S, Hendry GMA: Congenital absence of a lumbar pedicle. *Pediatr Radiol* 1982; 12:207.)

FIG 3–328.—A, simulated destruction of the pedicle on the right side of L-4 produced by scoliosis. B, tomogram shows pedicle to be intact.

FIG 3–329.—Posterior scalloping of the posterior aspects of the vertebral bodies may be seen as a normal variant, particularly in childhood. *Left,* 6-year-old. *Right,* 10-year-old.

FIG 3–330.—Posterior scalloping of the posterior aspects of the vertebral bodies in an asymptomatic 21-year-old man. This variation may also be seen in patients with spinal stenoses.

FIG 3–331.—The bodies of T-12 and L-1 are often slightly wedge-shaped and should not be mistaken for fractures. Note that both end-plates are angled and there is no condensation of bone or buckling anteriorly. (Ref: Lauridsen KN, et al: Degree of vertebral wedging of the dorsolumbar spine. *Acta Radiol Diagn* 1984; 25:29.)

FIG 3–332.—Another example of normal wedging of the bodies of T-12, L-1, and L-2.

FIG 3–333.—Long lumbar vertebrae.

FIG 3–334.—Oversized lumbar vertebra.

FIG 3–335.—Spurred osteoporotic vertebra may produce an appearance suggesting pathologic destruction. **A,** plain film. **B** and **C,** tomograms. (Ref: Wagner A: "Spurious" defect of the lumbar vertebral body. *AJR* 1980; 135:1095.)

FIG 3–336.—Multiple spurious defects of the lumbar spine in an 83-year-old woman.

FIG 3–337.—Hypertrophic spurring of the spinous processes may produce areas of relative radiolucency that might be mistaken for areas of bone destruction. Note also localized ossifications in the supraspinous and interspinous ligaments between the spinous processes, an aging phenomenon. (Refs: Jacobson HG, et al: The "swayback" syndrome. *AJR* 1958; 79:677; and Scapinelli R: Localized ossifications in the supraspinous and interspinous ligaments of adult man. *Rays (Rome)* 1988; 13:29.)

FIG 3–338.—Calcification of the interspinous ligament in an 81-year-old man. These calcifications are an aging phenomenon and should not be mistaken for an avulsion fracture. (Ref: Scapinelli R. Localized ossifications in the supraspinous and interspinous ligaments in adult man. *Rays (Rome)* 1988; 13:29.)

FIG 3–339.—A bone island of L-1. (Ref: Resnick D, Nemeek AA Jr, Haghighi P: Spinal enostoses (bone islands). *Radiology* 1983; 147:373.)

FIG 3–340.—Two examples of failure of union of the ossification centers of the tip of the spinous process of L-5

FIG 3–341.—Ununited secondary ossification center (limbus vertebra), simulating a fracture of L-5. **A,** plain film. **B,** laminagram. There is evidence to suggest that limbus vertebrae are the result of intravertebral disc herniation. (Ref: Kozlowski K: Anterior intravertebral disc herniations in children: Unrecognized chronic trauma to the spine. *Australas Radiol* 1979; 23:67.)

FIG 3–342.—Other examples of ununited secondary lumbar ossification centers (limbus vertebrae).

FIG 3–343.—The ring apophysis of L-5 seen in its entirety in an 8-year-old girl.

FIG 3–344.—Normal posterior "stepping" of lumbar vertebrae on extension (A). Normal alignment in neutral position (B).

FIG 3–345.—Wedge shape of L-5 and bowing of the inferior end-plates are normal variations and not reflections of pathology. (Ref: Frank DF, Miller JE: Hypoplasia of the lumbar vertebral body simulating spondylolisthesis. *Radiology* 1979; 133:59.)

FIG 3–346.—Apparent reverse spondylolisthesis of L-5 on S-1. The apparent displacement is usually due to errors in positioning. In some individuals, it results from the fact that the anteroposterior diameter of the superior surface of the sacrum is smaller than the inferior surface of the fifth lumbar vertebra. The anterior relationships are more reliable. (Ref: Melamed A, Ansfield DJ: Posterior displacement of lumbar vertebrae. *AJR* 1947; 58:307.)

FIG 3–347.—*Left*, apparent retrospondylolisthesis of L-5 on S-1 due to rotation. *Right*, true lateral shows normal relationships.

FIG 3–348.— Simulated defect produced by the neural arch of L-5. A CT scan showed a herniated nucleus but no defect in the vertebral body.

FIG 3–349.—Unilateral sacralization of L-5 on left side. Note the additional density created in the lateral projection. The anomalous articulation should not be mistaken for a fracture.

FIG 3–350.—Two other examples of anomalous articulations between L-5 and the sacrum. This anatomic arrangement is essentially unstable and may become symptomatic. (Ref: Jonsson B, et al: Anomalous lumbosacral articulations and low-back pain. *Spine* 1989; 14:831.)

FIG 3–351.—Anomalous articulation between the transverse process of L-5 and the adjacent sacrum.

FIG 3–352.—Patients with transitional vertebrae often have a significantly narrower lumbosacral disc than those with no transitional features. This narrowing does not imply disc degeneration. This finding is illustrated in this patient with 6 lumbar vertebrae. (Ref: Nicholson AA, et al: The measured height of the lumbosacral disc in patients with and without transitional vertebrae. *Br J Radiol* 1988; 61:454.)

FIG 3–353.—Conjoined lumbosacral nerve roots may be mistaken for the impressions of a disc herniation. Two root sleeves are demonstrated by metrizamide myelography. (Ref: Cail WS, Butler AB: Conjoined lumbosacral root sleeves. *Surg Neurol* 1983; 20:113.)

FIG 3–354.—Calcification of the iliolumbar ligament.

FIG 3–355.—An ununited ossification center for the superior articulating facet of S-1.

FIG 3–356.—Ununited ossification center for the spinous process of S-1.

FIG 3–357.—Calcification of the iliosacral ligaments.

FIG 3–358.—Accessory ossification centers for the sacral alae in a 15-year-old boy.

FIG 3–359.—"Angel-wing" sacrum, produced by calcification in the iliosacral ligaments.

FIG 3–360.—Calcification of the iliosacral ligament. Note simulation of destructive lesion in sacrum immediately below, produced by overlying colonic gas (⊣⊢).

FIG 3–361.—Unilateral anomalous articulation between S-1 and S-2.

FIG 3–362.—Simulated fracture of the sacrum in a young child. This appearance of the second and third sacral segments is not unusual in children.

FIG 3–363.—Normal variations in the appearance of the first sacral segment. **A,** normal relative increase in density in a 2-year-old boy. This is at times mistaken for osteosclerosis. **B,** pseudocyst of the sacrum *(arrow)* in a young adult due to the large amount of cancellous bone, with suggestion of a similar appearance in the second sacral segment.

FIG 3–364.—Widening of the posterior aspect of the S1–2 interspace, a variation in development in youth that may be mistaken for a destructive lesion. (Ref: Cacciarelli AA: Posterior widening of the S1–2 interspace in children: A normal variant of sacral development. *AJR* 1977; 129:305.)

FIG 3–365.—*Left*, the wide posterior aspect of the S1–2 interspace misdiagnosed as a fracture in a 13-year-old boy following paddling with a board. *Right*, follow-up film made 3 months later shows no change.

FIG 3–366.—The S1–2 posterior widening in a 15-year-old boy. At this age the end-plates are better defined.

FIG 3–367.—*Left,* lucency in posterior aspect of S-1 in a 16-year-old boy simulating a destructive lesion. *Right,* CT shows the shadows produced by normal trabeculation.

FIG 3–368.—Apparent cystic lesions of the sacrum, produced by the shadows of the fossae cribrosa of the sacrum. (Ref: Kreyenbühl W, Hessler C: A variation of the sacrum on the lateral view. *Radiology* 1973; 109:49.)

FIG 3–369.—A, simulated destructive lesion of S-1 due to rotation at time of filming. **B,** tomogram shows no abnormality.

FIG 3–370.—A, simulated destructive lesion of the sacrum produced by the fossae cribrosa and rotation. **B,** true lateral projection shows no abnormality.

FIG 3–371.—A, apparent fracture of the sacrum due to rotation at the time of filming. B, repeat film shows no abnormality.

FIG 3–372.—Large posterior elements of the fourth and fifth sacral segments.

FIG 3–373.—A, unusually deep sacral curve, which results in apparent expansile lesions with shell-like margins. B, CT shows no intrinsic lesion of the sacrum.

FIG 3–374.—Sacral ribs. A, unilateral. B, bilateral. C, bilateral and asymmetric sacral ribs. Note also calcification in iliolumbar ligaments (⟻) and ilial spur at the right sacroiliac joint (⊯). (Ref: Halloran W: Sacral ribs. *Q Bull Northwestern Univ Med School* 1960; 34:304.)

FIG 3–375.—Unilateral sacral rib also seen in lateral projection.

FIG 3–376.—Scoliosis of the sacrum and coccyx.

FIG 3–377.—Normal foraminal shadows in the sacrum.

FIG 3–378.—Simulated destructive lesions of the wings of the sacrum produced by the foramina of the sacrum. Bowel gas may accentuate this appearance as well. **A,** plain film. **B,** laminagram.

FIG 3–379.—Two examples of fossae in the sacral wings, simulating destructive lesions.

FIG 3–380.—Developmental variations in the sacrum. *Top left,* symmetric defects (→); *top right,* asymmetric defects (→). Calcification is present in the sacrospinal ligaments (↔). *Bottom,* other asymmetric defects.

FIG 3–381.—Normal poor definition of the sacroiliac joints in the adolescent. This appearance may at times simulate the changes of ankylosing spondylitis (see Fig 4–6).

FIG 3–382.—The alae of the sacral vertebrae in a 15-year-old boy.

FIG 3–383.—Three examples of secondary ossification centers of the wings of the sacrum.

FIG 3–384.—Unusual developmental cleft in the left side of the sacrum in a 9-year-old boy.

FIG 3–385.—Persistence of a secondary center of ossification of the sacrum in a 25-year-old woman.

FIG 3–386.—A, simulated obliteration of the sacroiliac joint due to slight rotation. This can be clarified by oblique projection of the sacroiliac joint (**B**).

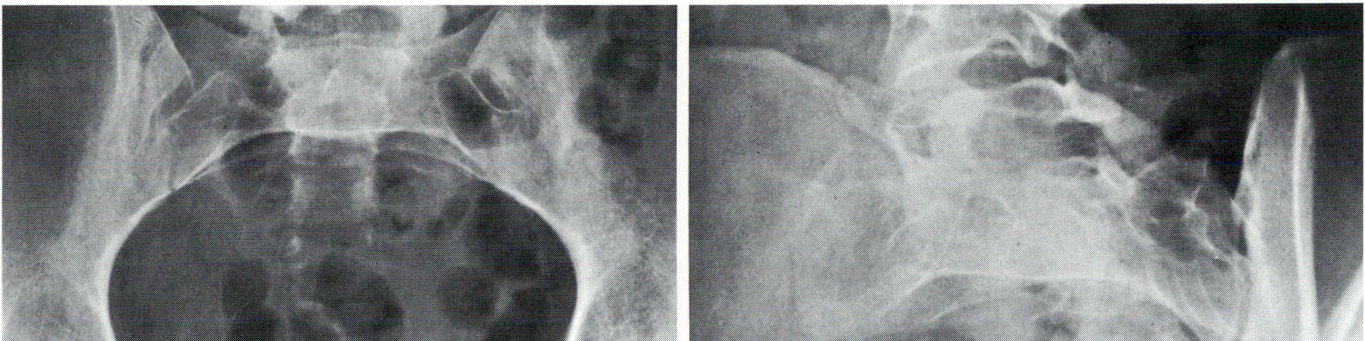

FIG 3–387.—*Left*, apparent absence of left sacroiliac joint due to differential plane of orientation of the joint compared with the patient's right side. *Right*, oblique projection shows an intact left sacroiliac joint.

FIG 3–388.—Two examples of bilateral accessory sacroiliac joints. (Ref: Ehara S, et al: The accessory sacroiliac joint: A common anatomic variant. *AJR* 1988; 150:857.)

FIG 3–389.—Vacuum phenomenon in the sacroiliac joints.

FIG 3–390.—Unilateral accessory sacroiliac joints that might be mistaken for fractures.

FIG 3–391.—Variations in development of the sacroiliac joints (*top*). CT sections illustrate the normal asymmetries to better advantage (*center* and *bottom*).

FIG 3–392.—Obliteration of the sacroiliac joints of the aged in a 73-year-old man. This phenomenon apparently may occur in the absence of inflammatory spondylitis. (Ref: Resnick D, et al: Clinical and radiographic abnormalities in ankylosing spondylitis: A comparison of men and women. *Radiology* 1976; 119:293.)

FIG 3–393.—Fusion lines of the sacral segments simulating fractures.

FIG 3–394.—Normal anterior angulation of the coccyx. The position of the coccyx is not useful, in itself, in the identification of trauma. (Ref: Postaccini F, Massolrio M: Idiopathic coccygodynia: Analysis of 51 operative cases and a radiographic study of the normal coccyx. *J Bone Joint Surg* 1983; 65A:1116.)

FIG 3–395.—Marked antiflexion of the coccyx.

FIG 3–396.—The ischial apophyses in a 15-year-old boy, not to be confused with a fracture of the tip of the coccyx.

FIG 3–397.—The junction of the coccyx and the last sacral segment mistaken for a fracture.

FIG 3–398.—Anterior angulation of the coccyx. Note portions of the posterior arch of the distal portion of the sacrum, which might be mistaken for fracture *(arrows)*.

FIG 3–399.—The ossification center for the first coccygeal segment in a 10-year-old child, which should not be confused with a calculus or enterolith.

FIG 3–400.—Congenital bifid coccyx.

FIG 3–401.—Congenital absence of the coccyx and anomalous development of the distal end of the sacrum.

The Pelvic Girdle

FIG 4–1.—Normal irregularity of the iliac crest in a 9-year-old boy. This appearance is typical before the development of the secondary ossification center for the crest of the ilium.

FIG 4–2.—"Double" iliac wings, produced by the shadow of the buttocks.

FIG 4–3.—Examples of the grooves for the nutrient arteries of the ilium.

FIG 4–4.—Normal lucency of the iliac fossae, which may resemble a cystic lesion in bone.

FIG 4–5.—Unusual fossae in the ilia in a 37-year-old man.

FIG 4–6.—Normal sclerosis and irregularity of the sacroiliac joints in a 14-year-old boy, resembling the changes of ankylosing spondylitis.

FIG 4–7.—Examples of preauricular (paraglenoidal) sulcus. This groove transmits the superior branch of the gluteal artery and supplies insertion for a portion of the sacroiliac ligament. It is apparently a characteristic of the female pelvis and is not necessarily symmetric (Ref: Dee PM: The preauricular sulcus. *Radiology* 1981; 140:354.)

FIG 4–8.—Unusual preauricular sulcus with asymmetry with opposite side.

FIG 4–9.—Small notches in the ilia adjacent to the sacroiliac joints in a 17-year-old boy.

FIG 4–10.—Developmental spurs at the inferior aspect of the sacroiliac joints. *Top left,* 30-year-old man. *Top right,* 30-year-old woman. *Bottom,* 55-year-old man.

FIG 4–11.—Crests for the insertion of the gluteus medius muscles. **A,** seen bilaterally. **B,** seen unilaterally and originally misinterpreted as a fracture.

FIG 4–12.—Irregular ossification of the ilium seen in adolescents, representing the origins of the sartorius muscle. These areas may mimic destructive lesions.

FIG 4–13.—The same entity as in Figure 4–12 with more localized radiolucencies.

FIG 4–14.—Spurring of muscle attachments at the ilium, seen in aged individuals.

FIG 4–15.—**A,** flanges on the edge of the ilium, which may simulate sclerotic lesions **(B).**

FIG 4–16.—Growing bone islands in a normal male. There is a 4-year interval between **A** and **B.** (Ref: Blank N, Lieber A: The significance of growing bone islands. *Radiology* 1965; 85:508.)

FIG 4–17.—Giant bone island in a 60-year-old man. (Refs: Smith J: Giant bone islands. *Radiology* 1973; 107:35; and Ehara S, et al: Giant bone island: Computed tomography findings. *Clin Imag* 1989; 13:231.)

FIG 4–18.—Iliac bone islands. **A,** a bone island in a 27-year-old man (←). These are common in the ilium, may grow, and occasionally disappear. They are of no clinical significance. A ring lesion (herniation pit) is present in the left femoral neck (⊬). **B,** growing bone island in a young woman. **C,** 9 years later, bone island has increased in size. (Ref: Kim SK, Barry WF Jr: Bone islands. *Radiology* 1968; 90:77.)

FIG 4–19.—Two examples of normal aging changes in the pelvic brim. This alteration in elderly patients may be mistaken for periostitis or Paget's disease (→). Note the normal spurring on the medial aspects of the obturator foramina (↠) in **A.**

FIG 4–20.—Ossification center for the anteroinferior iliac spine (←) and acetabular rim (⊩) in a 13-year-old boy.

FIG 4–21.—Prominent anteroinferior iliac spines in a 12-year-old boy.

FIG 4–22.—Two examples of pelvic "ears," a normal variant of development.

FIG 4–23.—**A,** irregularity of the anteroinferior iliac spine in an adolescent boy. This represents a "tug" lesion at the insertion of the rectus femoris muscle and should not be mistaken for the changes of neoplasm. **B,** enlargement of area of interest. Note that the muscle planes are not disturbed. (Ref: Murray RO, Jacobson HG: *The Radiology of Skeletal Disorders,* ed 2. New York, Churchill Livingstone, 1977, p 274.)

FIG 4–24.—Old healed "tug" lesions of the anteroinferior iliac spines.

FIG 4–25.—Combined pelvic "ears" (→) and healed "tug" lesions (↠) of the anteroinferior iliac spine in a 24-year-old man with pelvic fractures.

FIG 4–27.—An iliac rib (pelvic digit), a developmental anomaly. Note pseudoarticulation (←). (Ref: Greenspan A, Norman A: The "pelvic digit"—an unusual developmental anomaly. *Skeletal Radiol* 1982; 9:118.)

FIG 4–26.—Ring-like lesion of the ilium in a 31-year-old man. This is probably a developmental defect in bone and is of no clinical significance.

FIG 4–28.—Remnants of the synchondrosis between the ilium and ischium in a 12-year-old girl.

FIG 4–29.—Asymmetric closure of the synchondrosis between the ilium and ischium in an 8-year-old girl, misinterpreted as a fracture.

FIG 4–30.—Faulty positioning with rotation may simulate medial protrusion of the ischium and a fracture through the triradiate cartilage in a normal immature pelvis. **A,** infant. **B,** older child. (Ref: Shipley RT, et al: Artifact of projection simulating a pelvic fracture. *AJR* 1983; 141:479.)

FIG 4–31.—Double ossification centers of the pubis in a 3-month-old child. This appearance should not be mistaken for evidence of child abuse. (Ref: Caffey J, Madell SH: Ossification of the pubic bones at birth. *Radiology* 1956; 67:346.)

FIG 4–32.—Cephalad angulation of the beam may produce a double contour of the upper aspects of the superior pubic rami, which may be mistaken for periosteal proliferation. **A,** marked cephalad angulation. **B,** less cephalad angulation. **C,** perpendicular projection shows only a single contour of the bone.

FIG 4–33.—Simulated periosteal proliferation of the superior rami of the pubis in an 8-year-old due to cephalad angulation of the beam.

FIG 4–34.—Normal variations and asymmetry in closure of the ischiopubic synchondrosis. These are normal phenomena, which should not be mistaken for evidence of osteochondrosis.

FIG 4–35.—Incomplete development of the obturator rings in an otherwise healthy woman.

FIG 4–36.—Incomplete closure of the ischiopubic synchondrosis in a 72-year-old woman. Note accessory ossification centers in gaps *(arrows)*. (Ref: Sandomenico C, Tamburrini O: Bilateral accessory ossification center of the ischiopubic synchondroses in a female infant. *Pediatr Radiol* 1981; 10:253.)

FIG 4–37.—Failure of closure of the ischiopubic synchondrosis in a healthy 21-year-old woman.

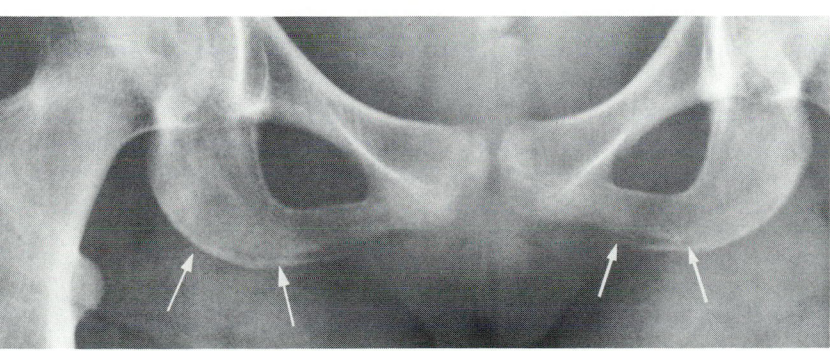

FIG 4–38.—The normal ischial apophyses in a 20-year-old woman.

FIG 4–39.—An unusual presentation of the ischial apophysis in the lateral projection of the hip in a 13-year-old boy. *Left*, AP view shows only the margin of the apophysis. *Right*, the apophysis seen in lateral projection of the hip.

FIG 4–40.—Prominent ischial apophysis in an asymptomatic 12-year-old boy.

FIG 4–41.—Normal irregularities of ossification of the ischia in adolescent children. These changes are usually asymmetric and disappear with increasing age. These alterations represent "tug" lesions due to the pull of the hamstring muscles on the apophyses.

FIG 4–42.—Remnant of the ischial apophysis in a 22-year-old woman.

FIG 4–43.—Fused ischial apophyses in a 26-year-old man.

FIG 4–44.—Simulated destructive lesion in the ischium due to edge of the ischial tuberosity. The same phenomenon is present to a lesser degree on the opposite side.

FIG 4–45.—Accessory ossification centers at the symphysis pubis. **A,** 19-year-old man. **B,** 20-year-old man.

FIG 4–46.—Ununited inferior pubic ossification centers in a 25-year-old woman.

FIG 4–47.—Normal irregular ridges on the medial aspects of the pubic bones in a 22-year-old man.

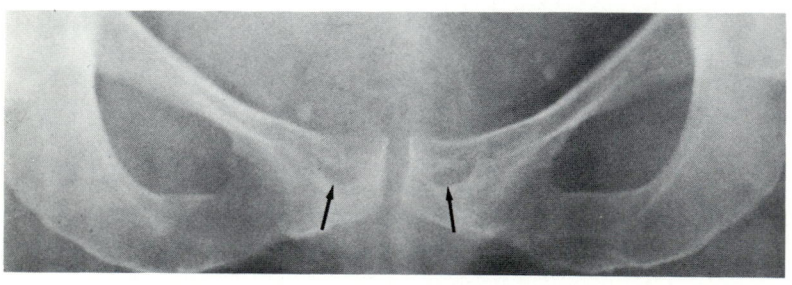

FIG 4–48.—Simulated cysts of the symphysis pubis produced by areas of thin bone below the superior ramus of the pubis.

FIG 4–50.—Normal irregularities of the margins of the symphysis pubis in a 12-year-old girl.

FIG 4–49.—Fossae in the inferior rami of the pubis.

FIG 4–51.—Postpartum changes in the symphysis pubis.

FIG 4–52.—Pubic spurs are a common normal variation in development. The malalignment of the symphysis in **A** is a postpartum alteration.

FIG 4–53.—Unilateral pubic spurs. The condensing changes about the symphysis and the irregularity of the symphyseal margins are postpartum changes.

FIG 4–54.—Ossification of the suprapubic ligament in a 42-year-old woman.

FIG 4–55.—Calcification of the suprapubic ligament in a 74-year-old man.

FIG 4–56.—Normal malalignment of the symphysis pubis in a 14-year-old girl. The lower margin of the symphysis is a more reliable indicator of the level than the upper margin. (Ref: Vix VA, Ryu CY: The adult symphysis pubis: Normal and abnormal. *AJR* 1971; 112:517.) Note also the accessory ossification center in the margin of the left side of the symphysis. Such accessory centers are common in the juvenile symphysis *(arrow)*.

FIG 4–57.—Normal malalignment and irregularities of the symphysis pubis in a 21-year-old woman.

FIG 4–58.—Normally wide symphysis pubis in an adolescent, a 12-year-old boy.

FIG 4–59.—Congenitally wide symphysis pubis in a young man with no history of trauma or developmental defect. This is a rare isolated variant. (Ref: Muecke EC, Currarino G: Congenital widening of the pubic symphysis: Associated clinical disorders and roentgen anatomy of affected bony pelves. *AJR* 1968; 103:179.)

FIG 4–60.—The ischial apophysis, seen en face, may simulate a fracture in adolescence.

FIG 4–61.—The ischial apophysis seen en face unilaterally.

FIG 4–62.—Postpartum symphyseal changes in the symphysis pubis with vacuum phenomenon.

FIG 4–63.—Spurs in the obturator foramen arising from the pubis, a finding usually seen in the elderly.

FIG 4–64.—Discrete radiolucencies in the ischia produced in part by the crossing shadow of the pubis. These are seen in children and adults.

The Pelvic Girdle—The Pubis and Ischium   **311**

FIG 4–65.—Normal protrusio acetabuli (←) in a 7-year-old girl. This is a normal phenomenon seen in children from about 4 to 12 years of age. Note also the normal radiolucent patches above the acetabula (⫢). (Ref: Alexander C: The aetiology of primary protrusio acetabuli. *Br J Radiol* 1965; 38:567.)

FIG 4–66.—Normal irregularity of the acetabular roofs in a young child. This appearance is normal between the ages of 7 and 12 years.

FIG 4–67.—Chondroid stripes in the acetabulum in a 12-year-old girl. This is a common finding in adolescents.

FIG 4–68.—Normal nutrient foramina, multiple on the patient's right and single on his left.

FIG 4–69.—Pit for nutrient vessels in acetabulum (←). If completely superimposed on the femoral head, this shadow may simulate a destructive lesion (⫢). **A,** plain film. **B,** laminagram.

FIG 4–70.—Accessory ossification centers in the superior portions of the acetabula (os acetabuli marginalis superior) in a 14-year-old boy (←). Note also additional ossification centers in the acetabula at lower level (⫢). These centers usually fuse solidly with the contiguous portions of the ilium. (Ref: Caffey J: *Pediatric X-ray Diagnosis,* ed 8. Chicago, Year Book Medical Publishers, 1985, p 331.)

FIG 4–71.—Accessory ossification centers (←) in a 14-year-old boy with additional centers laterally (⫢).

FIG 4–72.—Partial union of secondary ossification center of the acetabulum in the adolescent (←).

FIG 4–73.—Additional example of multiple accessory ossification centers of the acetabulum in a 14-year-old girl.

FIG 4–74.—An os acetabuli marginalis superior, persisting as a separate ossicle into adult life.

FIG 4–75.—An os acetabuli marginalis superior, persisting into adult life in a 22-year-old man.

The Pelvic Girdle—The Acetabulum   313

FIG 4–76.—Three examples of persistence of all or portions of secondary ossification centers of the acetabulum in adults. These may be mistaken for fractures.

FIG 4–77.—Incomplete closure of the os acetabuli marginalis superior producing apparent radiolucencies in the heads of the femurs in a 32-year-old man.

FIG 4–78.—Incomplete closure of the ossification centers of the acetabulum simulating fractures in a 40-year-old man.

FIG 4–79.—A, another example of the accessory center of ossification of the posterior lip of the acetabulum simulating a fracture in a 32-year-old woman. B, a similar but less marked appearance is present in opposite hip.

FIG 4–80.—Persistence of a secondary center of ossification of the posterior lip of the acetabulum, which was mistaken for a fracture. A, conventional film. B, tomogram.

FIG 4–81.—The same entity as in the preceding two figures with CT confirmation.

FIG 4–82.—Two examples of the os acetabuli, an accessory bone. This ossicle should be distinguished from calcification in the rectus femoris tendon insertion. (Ref: Kawashima A, et al: Paraacetabular periarthritis calcarea: Its radiographic manifestations. *Skeletal Radiol* 1988; 17:476.)

FIG 4–83.—A large accessory bone at the posterior margin of the acetabulum.

FIG 4–84.—Spur-like margins of the acetabulum (→). Note the ununited ossification center (⇸).

FIG 4–85.—**A,** the anterior lip of the acetabulum (→) and the posterior lip (↦) may be identified in most individuals. Between them, there is a relative radiolucency, best seen on the patient's right side. **B** and **C,** the lucent interval in these two patients produces an appearance simulating a fracture of the posterior wall of the acetabulum. (See also Figs 4–79 through 4–81.)

FIG 4–86.—Hypertrophic changes at the femoral head may produce an appearance simulating a fracture of the femoral neck.

FIG 4–87.— Apparent defects in the acetabulum due to projection and not anatomic alteration. (Ref: Kohler A, Zimmer EA: *Borderlands of the Normal and Early Pathologic in Skeletal Roentgenology,* ed 3. New York, Grune & Stratton, 1968, p 389.)

FIG 4–88.— Simulated destructive lesion of the acetabulum (←) due to an undulation in the anterior margin of the acetabulum coupled with superimposition of the shadow of the ischium (╫). This might be mistaken for a lesion on the apex of the acetabulum.

FIG 4–89.— Two other examples of fossae, which should not be mistaken for pathologic processes.

FIG 4–91.— A bone island in the acetabulum.

FIG 4–90.— In the lateral projection of the hip, the superior margin of the acetabulum may simulate a cyst.

FIG 4–92.— The roofs of the acetabula may project asymmetrically in normal individuals.

FIG 4–93.— The superior acetabular notch is the result of an accessory fossa in the apex of the acetabulum and is of no significance per se. (Ref: Johnstone WH, et al: The anatomic basis for the superior acetabular roof notch: "Superior acetabular notch." *Skeletal Radiol* 1982; 8:25.)

FIG 4–94.— Marked notching of the roof of the acetabulum.

FIG 4–95.— Unusual second lateral notch in the roof of the acetabulum in a young woman. (Courtesy of Dr. W.B. Guilford.)

FIG 4–96.—Two examples of asymmetric lateral acetabular notches, which are also probably due to fossae in the acetabulum.

FIG 4–97.—Normal triangular area of lucency above the acetabulum (→). This is normally symmetric bilaterally. The greater radiolucency is due to metastatic neoplasm (↦).

Chapter 5

The Shoulder Girdle and Thoracic Cage

FIG 5–1.—Normal appearance of the ossification centers of the coracoid processes in a 5-year-old boy.

FIG 5–2.—Normal appearance of the coracoid processes during growth. **A,** 13-year-old boy before appearance of the secondary ossification center. **B,** 15-year-old boy. Note secondary ossification centers for coracoid and acromion processes.

FIG 5–3.—Appearance of the ossification center of the coracoid process in adolescence before fusion occurs. It may be mistaken for a fracture. **A,** axillary projection. **B,** arm elevated.

FIG 5–5.—The synchondrosis of the base of the coracoid in a 15-year-old boy that simulates a cleft in the glenoid as seen in axillary projection.

FIG 5–4.—The apophysis of the coracoid process mistaken for a fracture in a 14-year-old boy.

FIG 5–6.—Normal irregularity of the growing glenoid processes in a 12-year-old boy.

FIG 5–7.—The ring apophysis of the glenoid fossa seen at anterior and posterior margins.

FIG 5–8.—The secondary apophysis of the tip of the coracoid process.

FIG 5–9.—Apparent lucencies in the neck of the scapula due to end-on projection of the coracoid (←). Note position of coracoid tip (↔).

FIG 5–10.—The coracoid process seen in the oblique projection of the shoulder.

FIG 5–11.—Secondary ossification centers for the glenoid, which should not be mistaken for fractures. (Ref: Ogden JA, Phillips SB: Radiology of postnatal skeletal development: VII. The scapula. *Skeletal Radiol* 1983; 9:157.)

FIG 5–12.—Secondary centers of ossification of the glenoid. Note the large apophysis at the superior margin.

FIG 5–13.—Failure of fusion of the apophysis at the superior margin of the glenoid in an adult.

FIG 5–14.—Small ossicle at the superior margin of the glenoid in an adult similar to that in Figure 5–13. This may be mistaken for calcific tendinitis of the long head of the biceps tendon. (Ref: Goldman AB: Calcific tendinitis of the long head of the biceps brachii distal to the glenohumeral joint. *AJR* 1989; 153:1011.)

FIG 5–15.—Ununited portion of the glenoid apophysis seen in the axial projections may be mistaken for a fracture fragment.

FIG 5–16.—Persistence of the glenoid apophysis in an adult.

FIG 5–17.—Small ossicle at margin of the glenoid fossa that may represent a remnant of the apophysis. *Left,* frontal projection. *Right,* axillary projection.

FIG 5–18.—Normal excrescences of the lower margin of the neck of the scapula, which may be mistaken for periostitis.

FIG 5–19.—Normal radiolucency of the wing of the scapula, which may resemble a cystic lesion.

FIG 5–20.—Sclerotic margins of the scapular fossae.

FIG 5–21.—Simulated fracture of the scapula by superimposition of the free margin of the scapula.

FIG 5–22.—Two examples of articulations between the scapula and adjacent ribs.

FIG 5–23.—Development of the acromion processes as separate centers in a 1-year-old girl.

FIG 5–24.—Unusually long and stout acromion processes in a 6-year-old boy.

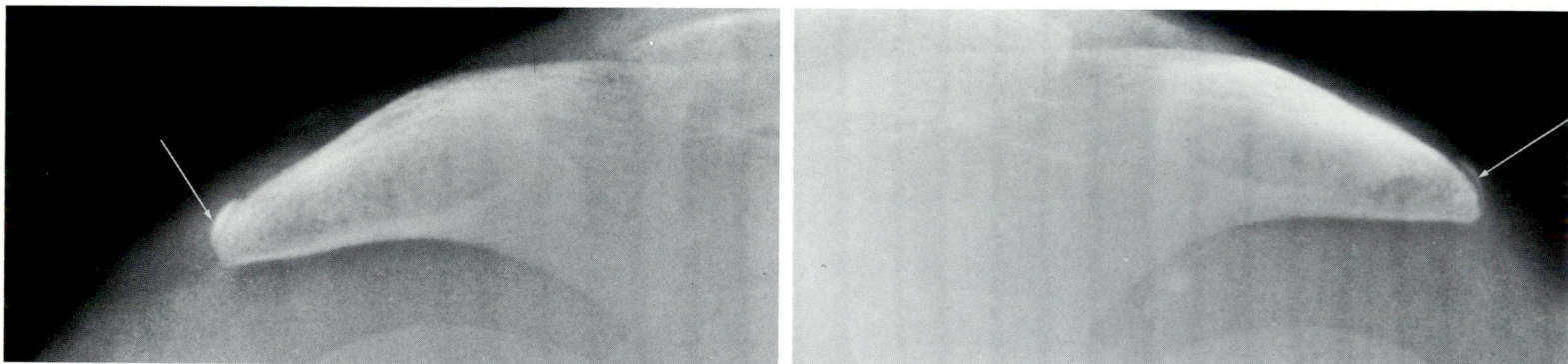

FIG 5–25.—The apophysis of the end of the acromion in a 16-year-old boy should not be mistaken for fracture.

FIG 5–26.—Persistent apophysis of the acromion in a 17-year-old boy. The opposite side was closed.

FIG 5–27.—Positioning of the arms in children may produce an appearance simulating acromioclavicular separation. **A,** external rotation. **B,** internal rotation.

FIG 5–28.—Variations in configuration of the acromioclavicular joint. **A,** in most normal individuals the inferior aspect of the clavicle is at the same level as the inferior aspect of the acromion. **B** and **C,** in a small percentage of normal individuals the distal end of the clavicle lies above or below the acromion (in this case above) and might be interpreted as an acromioclavicular separation. This variation emphasizes the value of examining both sides. (Refs: Urist MR: Complete dislocations of the acromioclavicular joint. *J Bone Joint Surg* 1946; 28:813; and Pettrone FA, Nirschl RP: Acromioclavicular dislocation. *Am J Sports Med* 1978; 6:160.)

FIG 5–29.—Another example of normal, but apparently dislocated, acromioclavicular joints. Note also the unusual width of the joint.

FIG 5–30.—Unusually wide acromioclavicular joints in a normal individual. These measurements exceed the quoted normal range. Examination of both shoulders will resolve this problem. (Ref: Petersson CJ, Redlund-Johnell I: Radiographic joint space in normal acromioclavicular joints. *Acta Orthop Scand* 1983; 54:431.)

FIG 5–31.—The normal closing acromial apophysis in a 13-year-old boy. The irregularity of the apophyseal line is normal.

FIG 5–32.—Normal closing acromial apophyses. Note the irregular mineralization and density of the center in **(B).**

FIG 5–33.—The apophysis of the acromion in a 14-year-old boy in axillary projection. This closes at 18 to 20 years of age.

FIG 5–34.—Remnant of line of closure of secondary ossification center for the acromion in an 18-year-old man.

FIG 5–35.—Two examples of the os acromiale. This secondary ossification center persists into adult life as a separate bone and is often mistaken for a fracture of the acromion process when seen in the axillary projection. It is usually, but not invariably, bilateral. (Ref: Fery A, Sommelet J: Os acromiale: Diagnosis, pathology and clinical significance. *French J Orthop Surg* 1988; 2:190).

FIG 5–36.—The os acromiale may occasionally be seen in the frontal projection *(left)* as well as in the axillary projection *(right)*.

FIG 5–37.—The os acromiale seen in the tangential view of the scapula.

FIG 5–38.—Normal fossa in the acromion process, simulating a destructive lesion.

FIG 5–39.—Normally wide acromioclavicular joint and apparent malalignment in a 14-year-old girl (←). This appearance, if not compared with the opposite side, may be mistaken for an acromioclavicular separation. Note also the secondary ossification center for the tip of the acromion process (⊬).

FIG 5–42.—An infrascapular bone simulating a rib fracture.

FIG 5–40.—Two examples of secondary ossification centers (infrascapular bone) of the inferior angle of the scapula in 16-year-old boys. These usually fuse by age 20 years.

FIG 5–41.—An infrascapular bone mistaken for a lung lesion.

FIG 5–43.—Hook-like configuration of the distal angles of the scapula.

FIG 5–44.—Unusual notch on the superior medial angles of the scapulae.

FIG 5–45.—Double cortical lines of the scapular spines in a 3-year-old child.

FIG 5–46.—Clasp-like cranial margin of the scapula, which produces a pseudoforamen. The thin sheet of bone that forms the fossa supraspinatus appears to be absent. (Ref: Goldenberg DB, Brogdon BG: Congenital anomalies of the pectoral girdle demonstrated by chest radiography. *J Can Assoc Radiol* 1967; 18:472.)

FIG 5–47.—Examples of calcification of the transverse superior ligament of the scapula. (Ref: Kohler A, Zimmer EA: *Borderlands of the Normal and Early Pathologic in Skeletal Roentgenology,* ed 3. New York, Grune & Stratton, 1968, p 156.)

FIG 5–48.—The superior end of the body of the scapula simulating a fracture fragment.

FIG 5–49.—Deep notch on the superior margin of the scapula (→). Note also partial formation of a coraco-clavicular articulation (↠) in **A.**

FIG 5–50.—Foramina-like defects in the superior border of the scapula.

FIG 5–51.—Two examples of developmental defects in the glenoid. These may be similar in origin to the acetabular notch (see Fig 4–93).

FIG 5–52.—Normal lucencies in the neck of the scapula that may be mistaken for destructive lesions. They probably represent the lucency of the cancellous bone of the glenoid marginated by the coracoid process.

FIG 5–53.—Striking example of the entity shown in Figure 5–52, mistaken for a true lesion. Note that it is not seen on the straight frontal projection *(top right)*.

FIG 5–54.—Developmental defects of the scapula that may be mistaken for a pathologic process. (Refs: Cigtay OS, Mascatello VJ: Scapular defects: A normal variation. *AJR* 1979; 132:239; and Pate D, et al: Scapular foramina. *Skeletal Radiol* 1985; 14:270.)

FIG 5–55.—Simulated fracture of the neck of the scapula, produced by trabecular pattern.

FIG 5–56.—Fat stripe of chest wall, simulating fracture of the scapula.

FIG 5–57.—Large nutrient foramen of the scapula.

FIG 5–58.—Two examples of vascular channels that might be mistaken for fracture.

FIG 5–59.—Vascular groove in the neck of the scapula.

FIG 5–60.—Prominent vascular channel in the wing of the scapula.

FIG 5–61.—Tangential views of the scapula with simulated fractures produced by the overlapping shadow of the free border on the body of the scapula.

FIG 5–62.—Examples of the normal "vacuum" phenomenon in the shoulder joint.

FIG 5–63.—"Vacuum" phenomenon in both shoulder joints. When the lucency is seen overlying only bone, as in **B**, it may be mistaken for fracture.

FIG 5-64.—Dysplastic scapulae with wide acromioclavicular joints and large shallow glenoid fossae. (Ref: Resnick D, et al: Bilateral dysplasia of the scapular neck. *AJR* 1982; 139:387.)

FIG 5-65.—Conventional positioning of the arms for chest radiography may produce an appearance simulating dislocations of the shoulders in children.

FIG 5-66.—*Left,* simulated dislocation of the right shoulder secondary to positioning in an elderly individual. *Right,* repeat examination shows improved relationships.

FIG 5-67.—Normal irregular appearance of the medial ends of the clavicles in an 18-year-old man. This appearance, before completion of development, may be misinterpreted as evidence of disease. **A,** plain film. **B,** laminagram.

FIG 5–68.—Secondary ossification centers of the medial ends of the clavicles in a 20-year-old man.

FIG 5–69.—Asymmetric closure of secondary ossification centers of medial ends of clavicles in a 21-year-old man. **A,** open apophysis (→). **B,** closed apophysis. Note also deep rhomboid fossa in **A** (↠).

FIG 5–70.—Failure of the medial ends of the clavicles to develop completely in an otherwise normal adult.

FIG 5–71.—An ununited ossification center for the medial end of the clavicle, which has persisted as a separate ossicle. Note cupped juvenile configuration of the adjacent end of the clavicle in contrast to the opposite side.

FIG 5–72.—Normal asymmetry of the medial ends of the clavicles.

FIG 5–73.—An accessory ossicle at the medial end of the clavicle.

FIG 5–74.—Simulated fracture of the medial end of the clavicle produced by overlapping shadows of the transverse processes, rhomboid fossa, and ribs.

FIG 5–75.—A dense closed epiphyseal line in an adult, simulating a fracture with overriding.

FIG 5–76.—Sclerosis of the medial ends of the clavicle in a healthy 41-year-old man.

FIG 5–77.—Unusually stout medial ends of the clavicles with cupping of the articular surfaces.

FIG 5–78.—Three examples of unilateral bifid medial ends of the clavicle.

FIG 5–79.—Two examples of the canal for the middle supraclavicular nerve.

FIG 5–80.—The nutrient channel of the clavicle is usually located posteriorly and not seen, but may appear on the inferior (**A**) or superior (**B**) borders. These may be mistaken for incomplete fractures. (Ref: Ogden JA, et al: Radiology of postnatal skeletal development: III. The clavicle. *Skeletal Radiol* 1979; 4:196.)

FIG 5–81.—The nutrient vessel of the clavicle mistaken for fracture in a 70-year-old man.

FIG 5–82.—The nutrient vessel of the clavicle, mistaken for a fracture in a 5-year-old boy.

FIG 5–83.—The nutrient vessel of the clavicle, mistaken for a fracture in a 43-year-old man.

FIG 5–84.—Examples of rhomboid fossae, the site of attachment of the rhomboid ligament between the first rib and the clavicle. Note how it may simulate bone destruction and the fact that it is not necessarily bilaterally symmetric.

FIG 5–85.—Rhomboid fossae, which could be mistaken for cavitary lesions in lung.

FIG 5–86.—Bilateral rhomboid fossae simulating apical pneumo-thoraces.

FIG 5–87.—Grooves for the insertion of the coracoclavicular ligament.

FIG 5–88.—Groove for the coracoclavicular ligament simulating an erosion.

FIG 5–89.—Groove for the insertion of the coracoclavicular ligament mistaken for a fracture. *Left,* external rotation. *Right,* internal rotation.

FIG 5–90.—Examples of deep fossae in the distal portions of the clavicle probably representing the origin of the deltoid muscle.

FIG 5–91.—Examples of wavy inferior margins of the clavicles thought to be related to the subclavian arteries. *Top,* bilateral. *Bottom,* unilateral on the right. It has also been suggested that this configuration may be the product of rotation of the clavicle with aging. (Refs: Levin B: The unilateral wavy clavicle. *Skeletal Radiol* 1990; 19:519; Freiberger RH: Letter to the editor. *Skeletal Radiol* 1990; 20:192.)

FIG 5–92.—Abortive articulations between the clavicle and the first rib.

FIG 5–93.—Three examples of the coracoclavicular joint, an anomalous articulation that develops in the coracoclavicular ligament and is usually of no clinical significance. (Refs: Cockshott WP: The coracoclavicular joint. *Radiology* 1973; 131:313; and Chen YM, Bohrer SP: Coracoclavicular and coracoacromial ligament calcification. *Skeletal Radiol* 1990; 19:263.)

FIG 5-94.—Developing coracoclavicular articulation in a 9-year-old child.

FIG 5-95.—Calcifications in the coracoclavicular ligament.

FIG 5-96.—The costoclavicular joint, an anomalous articulation between the clavicle and the anterior aspect of the first rib. (Ref: Redlund-Johnell I: The costoclavicular joint. *Skeletal Radiol* 1986: 15:25.)

FIG 5-97.—Unusual appearance of the clavicle, produced by overlapping shadow of the scapula.

FIG 5-98.—Unusually stout clavicular shafts in contrast to the medial and distal portions.

FIG 5-99.—Irregular appearance of the distal end of the clavicle before growth is completed in a 16-year-old.

FIG 5–100.—Simulated fracture of the distal end of the clavicles produced by a bony flange. **A,** plain film. **B,** tomogram.

FIG 5–101.—Large distal ends of the clavicle may have a "cyst-like" appearance due to the large amount of cancellous bone.

FIG 5–102.—An accessory ossicle in the acromioclavicular joint.

FIG 5–103.—Duplication of the distal end of the clavicle. (Ref: Twig HL,. Rosenbaum RC: Duplication of the clavicle. *Skeletal Radiol* 1981; 6:281.)

FIG 5–104.—Unusual duplication anomaly of the distal end of the clavicle.

FIG 5–105.—There is wide normal variation in the alignment of the acromion and the clavicle. The inferior margin of the clavicle aligns with the lower margin of the acromion in 81% of patients. The clavicle projects above the acromion in 7%, below the acromion in 7%, and overrides the acromion in 5%. Both sides should be examined routinely to detect these variations. *Top,* bilateral cephalad position of distal ends of the clavicles in relationship to the acromion. *Bottom,* very marked example of the same entity. (Ref: Keats TE, Pope TL: The acromioclavicular joint: Normal variation and diagnosis of dislocation. *Skeletal Radiol* 1988; 17:159.)

FIG 5–106.—Bilateral caudad position of the distal ends of the clavicles in relationship to the acromion.

FIG 5–108.—Duplication of the ossification centers of the lower portion of the body of the sternum in an 11-month-old child.

FIG 5–107.—Variations in development of the sternum. **A,** and **B,** accessory ossification centers for the body of the sternum in a 5-month-old girl. These, as well as duplication of the manubrial centers, may be seen in the lateral projection. (Ref: Ogden JA, et al: Radiology of postnatal skeletal development: II. The manubrium and sternum. *Skeletal Radiol* 1979; 4:189.)

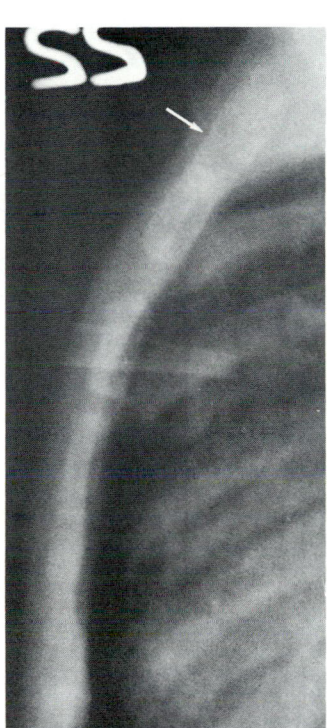

FIG 5–109.—Double ossification center of the manubrium in a normal 5-month-old boy. This is frequently seen in Down's syndrome but also occurs as a normal variant.

FIG 5–110.—The sternal ossification centers superimposed on the ribs in a badly positioned chest film, simulating healing rib fractures.

FIG 5–112.—Nonsegmentation of the sternum in a 30-yer-old man, probably secondary to premature fusion of centers.

FIG 5–111.—Variations in development of the sternum. **A,** development of the body of the sternum from only two centers. **B,** marked variability in size of the centers of ossification of the body of the sternum.

FIG 5–113.—Three examples of episternal processes.

FIG 5–114.—Examples of episternal bones in adults. (Refs: Brown WH: Episternal bones. *Radiology* 1960; 75:116; and Stark P, et al: Episternal ossicles. *Radiology* 1987; 165:143.)

FIG 5–115.—The manubrium in adults resembling mediastinal masses. Note in **A** the sclerosis of the borders of the manubrium, which may suggest a mass lesion with a calcified border.

FIG 5–116.—The manubrium in an 11-month-old child, mistaken for a mediastinal mass.

FIG 5–117.—Developmental irregularity of the superior margin of the sternum at the sternomanubrial joint in an adolescent boy. Defects of this type have been likened to Schmorl's nodes of the spine. (Ref: Kohler A, Zimmer EA: *Borderlands of the Normal and Early Pathologic in Skeletal Roentgenology*, ed 3. New York, Grune & Stratton, 1968, p 169.)

FIG 5–118.—The sternomanubrial joint may simulate a fracture of the dorsal spine in the frontal plane.

FIG 5–119.—Congenital bifid sternum, an unusual variant. Note the radiolucency in the midline in the frontal chest film (→) and the mass effect in the lateral film (⇢). (Courtesy of Dr. W. P. Brown.) (Ref: Larsen LL, Ibach HF: Complete congenital fissure of the sternum. *AJR* 1962; 87:1062.)

FIG 5–120.—Partial bifid sternum with union at distal end. (Courtesy of Dr. W. E. Litterer.)

FIG 5–121.—Two examples of sternal foramina, a finding of no significance. (Ref: Resnik CS, Brower AC: Midline circular defect of the sternum. *Radiology* 1979; 130:657.)

FIG 5–122.—Variations in configuration of the xiphoid process and calcified costal cartilage, simulating destructive or neoplastic lesions of the sternum, particularly if there are symptoms referable to this area. (From Keats TE: Four normal anatomic variations of importance to radiologists. *AJR* 1957; 78:89. Reproduced with permission.)

FIG 5–123.—**A,** plain film. Simulated mass lesion of the sternum produced by the xiphoid process and calcified costal cartilage (→). **B,** laminagram. Note posterior curvature of the xiphoid process, which contributes to this midleading appearance (↠).

FIG 5–124.—The normal junction of the xiphoid process and body of the sternum, not to be mistaken for a fracture.

FIG 5–125.—Indentation on anterior surface of the last sternal segment.

FIG 5–126.—Marked anterior flexion of the xiphoid process.

FIG 5–127.—Bifid xiphoid process.

FIG 5–128.—Bifid xiphoid process with one limb directed anteriorly.

FIG 5–129.—Elongated xiphoid process directed anteriorly. This type of xiphoid may be jointed as well. The anterior direction may produce an apparent epigastric mass on clinical examination. (Ref: Sanders PC, Knight RW: Radiologic appearance of the xiphoid process presenting as an upper abdominal mass. *Radiology* 1981; 141:489.)

FIG 5–130.—Accessory center (←) for the xiphoid process (↔).

FIG 5–131.—Unusual partitioned xiphoid processes.

FIG 5–132.—Simulated cupping of the anterior ends of the ribs produced by lordotic projection.

FIG 5–133.—Cervical rib in a 2-week-old infant.

FIG 5–134.—Accessory rib elements at transverse process of T-1.

FIG 5–135.—Well-developed cervical ribs in an adult.

FIG 5–136.—Jointed ligamentous calcifications between the transverse process of T-1 and the first rib.

FIG 5–137.— Cervical rib articulating at its distal end with an additional bony element.

FIG 5–138.—Large bilateral cervical ribs, which articulate with the first ribs.

FIG 5–140.—The anterior end of a cervical rib simulates a parenchymal lesion.

FIG 5–139.—This patient presented with a hard right supraclavicular mass, which is explained by the anomalous arrangement of the first and second ribs. Such variants may efface the supraclavicular fossa and simulate a mass. (Ref: Fakhry SM, Thomas CG Jr: Pseudotumor of the supraclavicular fossa. *South Med J* 1986; 79:822.)

FIG 5–142.—Developmental absence of the first rib. Note that the costal cartilages have formed even in the absence of the rib *(arrows).*

FIG 5–141.—Failure of first ribs to join costal cartilages.

FIG 5–143.—Three examples of anomalous articulations in the midportion of the first ribs, simulating a fracture (↔).

FIG 5–144.—Anomalous articulation in the first ribs, simulating a fracture in **A** and a mass lesion in **B**.

FIG 5–145.—Anomalous articulations in the left first rib.

FIG 5–146.—Two examples of normal areas of lucency in the anterior ends of the first ribs. These may be unilateral or bilateral, are fairly constant in their location, and should not be confused with areas of bone destruction.

FIG 5–147.—Developmental spurs at the costovertebral junctions.

FIG 5–148.—Ossicles related to rib ends. **A,** anterior rib end; **B,** posterior rib end.

FIG 5–149.—The costoclavicular joint. This joint is a variant of the ligamentous connection between the medial end of the clavicle and the first rib. (From Redlund-Johnell I: The costoclavicular joint. *Skeletal Radiol* 1986; 15:25. Used by permission.)

FIG 5–150.—Articulation between the first and second ribs.

FIG 5–151.—Spur-like process arising from the anterior portion of the first rib.

FIG 5–152.—Fusion of the anterior portions of the first and second ribs.

FIG 5–153.—Anomalous development of the anterior end of the fourth rib.

FIG 5–154.—Localized developmental fusions of portions of the posterior ribs may simulate parenchymal lesions or pneumothorax.

FIG 5–155.—Developmental fusion between the anterior ends of the first and second ribs.

FIG 5–156.—Fusions of the posterior portions of the right fifth, sixth, and seventh ribs, which can be seen in the lateral projection as well.

FIG 5–157.—Fusion of the posterior portion of the fourth and fifth ribs in a 12-year-old boy.

FIG 5–158.—Extensive developmental fusions of the posterior ribs.

FIG 5–159.—Normal exaggeration of the curve of the necks of the ribs, simulating rib notching.

FIG 5–160.—Marked cephalad angulation of the fourth ribs with fusion to the adjacent third ribs.

FIG 5–161.—Grooves in the lower margins of the ribs, which might be mistaken for the lung edge of a pneumothorax.

FIG 5–162.—Two examples of pseudoerosion of the ribs. Loss of bone from the superior aspects of the ribs may be seen in a variety of pathologic processes, particularly in connective tissue diseases, but may also be seen in normal individuals with increasing age. (Ref: Keats TE: Superior marginal rib defects in restrictive lung disease. *AJR* 1975; 124:449.)

FIG 5–163.—Two examples of simulated destruction of the inferior aspects of the posterior portions of the middle ribs. This variation is commonly seen and is due to the thin flange of bone at the lower portions of these ribs.

FIG 5–164.—Simulated "cysts" of proximal rib ends due to cancellous bone.

FIG 5–165.—Localized protuberances on the anterior aspects of the second and third ribs.

FIG 5–166.—Enlarged costovertebral articulations due to hypertrophic changes.

FIG 5–167.—Normal exaggeration of curvature of the necks of the lower ribs.

FIG 5–168.—Companion shadows along lower rib margins produced by thin bony flanges.

FIG 5–169.—Articulation between two ribs.

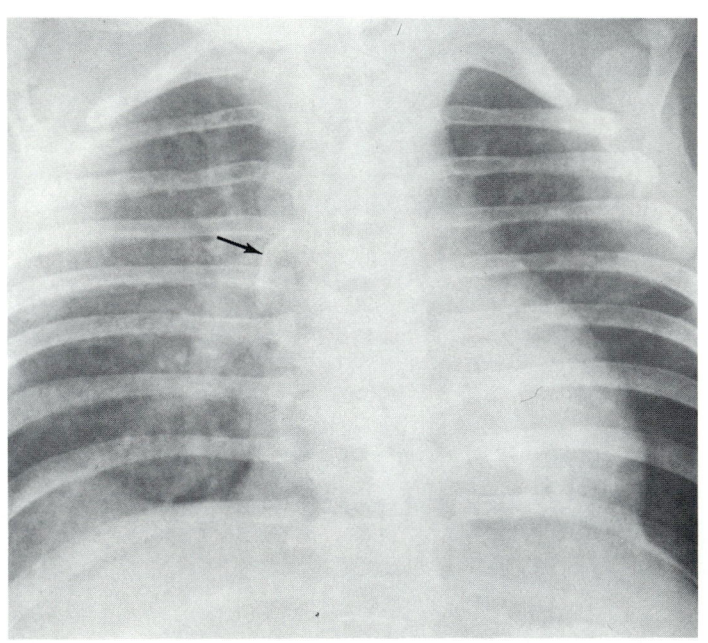

FIG 5–170.—Intrathoracic rib. A rare anomaly of no clinical significance. (Ref: Weinstein AS, Mueller CF: Intrathoracic rib. *AJR* 1965; 94:587.)

FIG 5–171.—Two additional examples of intrathoracic ribs.

FIG 5–172.—Intra-abdominal rib.

FIG 5–173.—Anomalous development of the twelfth ribs.

FIG 5–174.—A, duplication of the left eleventh rib. B, these ribs take a marked intra-abdominal course.

FIG 5–175.—Unilateral development of the twelfth rib.

FIG 5–176.—Unilateral development of the twelfth rib, simulating a fracture (→). Note the elongated transverse process on the opposite side (↦).

FIG 5–177.—Gastric contents, simulating sclerotic lesion of the rib.

FIG 5–178.—Anterior rib ends, simulating nodular lesions in lung.

FIG 5–179.—Two examples of the spinal laminae, simulating a pulmonary nodule. (Ref: Shortsleeve MJ, Foster SC: Pulmonary pseudonodule. *Radiology* 1979; 131:311.)

FIG 5–180.—Transverse process in cross-section, simulating cavitary lung lesion.

FIG 5–181.—Very large calcified costal cartilages simulate an intrathoracic lesion in both projections. **A** and **B,** a 74-year-old man. **C** and **D,** a 58-year-old man. The first sternocostal joint may be classified as either a synchondrosis or a synostosis, but a joint cavity lateral to the first sternocostal joint may be present. (Ref: Schils JP, et al: Sternocostal joints: Anatomic, radiographic and pathologic features in adult cadavers. *Invest Radiol* 1989; 24:596.)

FIG 5–182.—Very large hypertrophied costal cartilage of the first ribs with marked intrathoracic extension seen in lateral projection.

FIG 5–183.—Anomalous development of the first rib (→) with the costal cartilage ununited to the rib (→).

FIG 5–184.—Bilateral failure of the first costal cartilages to unite with the first rib.

FIG 5–185.—Large first rib with bifurcated anterior end mistaken for a mass lesion. *Left,* plain film. *Right,* tomogram.

FIG 5–186.—Variations in development of the costal cartilages of the first ribs.

FIG 5–187.—Extensive costal cartilage calcification in a 41-year-old man.

FIG 5–188.—Ring-shaped costal cartilage calcification simulating cavitary lesion in lung.

FIG 5–189.—Circular costal cartilage calcification, suggesting cavitary lesions in lung.

FIG 5–190.—Calcified costal cartilage misinterpreted as a metastatic deposit. The cartilage is jointed (←). *Left,* frontal projection. *Right,* oblique projection.

FIG 5–191.—Costal cartilage calcification, simulating vascular calcification.

FIG 5–192.—Linear costal cartilage calcification overlying the left kidney may be mistaken for a renal calculus.

Chapter 6

The Upper Extremity

FIG 6–1.—Bilateral duplicated capital humeral epiphyses in a 13-month-old child.

FIG 6–2.—Simulated aseptic necrosis of the humeral head in an elderly patient, produced by overlapping of the shadows of the humeral head and scapula. Note variation in width of dense area with changes in position of the shoulder. This appearance is accentuated by rotator cuff tear.

FIG 6–3.—Two examples of simulated periostitis produced by the shadow of the bicipital groove in neonates, seen with the arm externally rotated or elevated.

FIG 6–4.—Deep bicipital grooves, which may be mistaken for abnormality. **A,** 7 months old. **B,** 2 years old.

FIG 6–5.—The shadows of the bicipital groove in the adult. *Left,* external rotation. *Right,* internal rotation.

FIG 6–6.—Spur-like excrescences of the humeral metaphyses in an 82-year-old man. These are not uncommon in the elderly and may represent a "tug" lesion of the joint capsule.

FIG 6–7.—Metaphyseal spurs in a 19-month-old child. These appear to be normal variants of growth.

FIG 6–8.—Beaking of the epiphyseal line in a 16-year-old boy. This beaking, particularly of the epiphysis, is seen elsewhere and should not be mistaken for an avulsion injury (see Figs 6–119, 6–239, and 6–241). (From Keats TE, Harrison RB: The epiphyseal spur. *Skeletal Radiol* 1980; 5:175. Reproduced with permission.)

FIG 6–9.—Metaphyseal spur in a 13-year-old boy.

FIG 6–10.—The normal epiphyseal lines of the proximal humerus in a 17-year-old boy. **A,** external rotation; **B,** internal rotation. The epiphyseal line in **B** at times is mistaken for a fracture.

FIG 6–11.—Residuals of the closing epiphyseal line in a 16-year-old boy.

FIG 6–12.—The closed epiphyseal line in an 18-year-old man that simulates a lesion on CT.

FIG 6–13.—Bilateral upper humeral notches in an 11-year-old boy. These are seen in children between the ages of 10 and 16 years and represent a phase of growth. They are probably similar to the cortical lesions seen in the distal humerus, the distal end of the radius, the distal end of the femur, and the proximal end of the tibia (see Figs 6–52, 6–111, 7–100, 7–101, 7–110, and 7–218). (Ref: Ozonoff MB, Zeiter FM Jr: The upper humeral notch: A normal variant in children. *Radiology* 1974; 113:699.)

FIG 6–14.—Other examples of upper humeral notches. **A** and **A′**, 12-year old boy. **B** and **B′**, 14-year-old girl. Note how these variants may resemble the changes of malignancy.

FIG 6–15.—Upper humeral notch in a 13-year-old boy (←). Note also benign cortical defect (↤) and normal glenoid irregularities (⫢).

FIG 6–16.—Very deep upper humeral notch in a 7-year-old boy.

FIG 6–17.—Unusual ossicle at the upper end of the humerus.

FIG 6–18.—A, simulated impaction fracture of the humeral head seen in film made in internal rotation in a postictal patient. B, external rotation—normal.

FIG 6–19.—A, simulated fracture of the greater tuberosity produced by positioning in external rotation. B, no fracture seen with internal rotation.

FIG 6–20.—Two examples of how projection of the cortex of the humeral neck can simulate periostitis.

FIG 6–21.—Examples of simulated destruction of the greater tuberosity. This normal finding appears to represent the fusion line of the lateral portion of the epiphysis. Its position in relationship to the epiphyseal line should help differentiate it from a true lesion. (Ref: Resnick D, Cone RO: The nature of humeral pseudocysts. *Radiology* 1984; 150:27.)

FIG 6–22.—Bilateral visualization of the rotator cuff by surrounding fat in a 29-year-old man.

FIG 6–23.—Cortical thickening underlying the deltoid muscle insertions in a 2-month-old child.

FIG 6–24.—The insertion of the deltoid muscle in a 20-month-old child, which may simulate periostitis.

FIG 6–25.—Prominent deltoid muscle insertion in two projections in a 50-year-old man (→). The medial shadow in **A** is a soft tissue fold (⇸).

FIG 6–26.—Deltoid muscle insertions that resemble periostitis.

FIG 6–27.—Localized cortical thickenings due to a prominent deltoid muscle insertion.

FIG 6–28.—Radiolucencies produced by the insertion of the pectoralis major muscle. **A,** plain film. **B,** laminagraphy. (From Brower AC: Cortical defect of the humerus at the insertion of the pectoralis major. *AJR* 1977; 128:677. Used by permission.)

FIG 6–29.—The same entity as in Figure 6–28 seen bilaterally in a heavily muscled 19-year-old man.

FIG 6–30.—Cortical thickenings of the medial and posterior cortex at insertion of the latissimus dorsi muscle in a 55-year-old man.

FIG 6–31.—Latissimus dorsi muscle insertions in a 68-year-old man with endocortical thickenings.

FIG 6–32.—Spur-like insertion of latissimus dorsi muscle.

FIG 6–33.—A, benign cortical defects of the humerus in a 4-year-old child (←). Note also the location and appearance of the ossification centers for the greater tuberosity and head of the humerus at this age (⊹). **B,** 5 years later, the cortical defect in the left humerus has disappeared; that on the right has left a sclerotic scar.

FIG 6–34.—Multiple benign cortical defects of the proximal humerus. These fibrous lesions may be single or multiple and are of no clinical significance. (Ref: Caffey J: *Pediatric X-Ray Diagnosis*, ed 8. Chicago, Year Book Medical Publishers, 1985, p 446.)

FIG 6–35.—Two examples of "herringbone" trabecular pattern of the medullary cavity of the humerus.

FIG 6–36.—**A** and **B**, a 26-year-old woman with "herringbone" medullary pattern of her left humerus. **C**, her right humerus 2 weeks after casting for fracture of the surgical neck. Note the peculiar type of deossification, which occurs in patients with this type of medullary trabecular pattern and resembles metastatic neoplasm or multiple myeloma. (Ref: Keats TE, Harrison RB: A pattern of posttraumatic demineralization of bone simulating permeative neoplastic replacement. *Skeletal Radiol* 1978; 3:113.) On close inspection this type of aggressive osteoporosis will show small cortical lucencies that will help differentiate it from malignant neoplastic permeation. (Ref: Helms CA, Munk PL: Pseudopermeative skeletal lesions. *Br J Radiol* 1990; 63:461.)

FIG 6–37.—Two examples of physiologic "periostitis" of the newborn. **A,** 3-month-old infant. **B,** 8-month-old infant. This is not seen before age 1 month and is usually symmetric in distribution, although not necessarily concentric, and may be seen in only one view. (Ref: Shopfner CE: Periosteal bone growth in normal infants: A preliminary report. *AJR* 1966; 97:154.)

FIG 6–38.—Normal thin flange of bone above the lateral epicondyle, which simulates periostitis (←). Note also the perforated olecranon fossa (⧻).

FIG 6–39.—Simulated periostitis produced by the lateral epicondylar flange in another individual.

FIG 6–40.—The epicondylar flange simulating a cortical fracture.

FIG 6–41.—Olecranon foramen with marked sclerosis of its margins.

FIG 6–42.—The supracondylar process. This vestigial structure is rarely associated with symptoms and occurs in about 1% of persons of European origin. Its axis is typically directed distally. (Ref: Barnard LB, McCoy SM: The supracondyloid process of humerus. *J Bone Joint Surg* 1946; 28:845.)

FIG 6–43.—The supracondylar process in a 4-year-old boy.

FIG 6–44.—A supracondylar process directed cephalad rather than in the usual caudad direction.

FIG 6–45.—Developmental cortical notch on the medial cortex, of no significance. Its anatomic origin is uncertain.

FIG 6–46.—Another example of the humeral cortical notch.

FIG 6–47.—Developmental foramen above the medial epicondyle. Note its similarity to the notch in Figure 6–46.

FIG 6–48.—Variations in appearance of the olecranon fossa. **A,** the fossa is replaced by a complete foramen (←). **B,** the foramen is traversed by a bridge of bone (⊹).

FIG 6–49.—Simulated supratrochlear foraminal bone or fracture produced by the ossification center for the olecranon process in a 7-year-old girl.

FIG 6–50.— The normal rarefaction of bone of the distal humerus may simulate a cystic lesion in the lateral projection.

FIG 6–51.— Simulated fractures produced by soft tissue folds.

FIG 6–52.— Apparent discontinuity of bone immediately above the epiphyseal line in a 12-year-old boy. This represents a variation in development of the metaphysis of a long bone in adolescence similar to the cortical lesions seen in the proximal end of the humerus, the distal radius, the distal end of the femur, and the proximal end of the tibia. This appearance may be misconstrued as evidence of dislocation of the epiphysis or a destructive lesion of the humerus (see Figs 6–13, 6–111, 7–100, 7–101, 7–110, 7–218). (Ref: Silberstein MJ, et al: Some vagaries of the capitellum. *J Bone Joint Surg* 1979; 61A:244.)

FIG 6–53.— The discontinuity seen in Figure 6–52 is now only minimally present in this 16-year-old boy, indicating the transient nature of this finding.

FIG 6–54.—Early appearance of the ossification center for the trochlea in a 6-year-old girl. Rarely the trochlear ossification may appear without evidence of a medial epicondylar center as in this case. (Ref: Resnik CS, Hartenberg MA: Ossification centers of the pediatric elbow: A rare normal variant. *Pediatr Radiol* 1986; 16:254.)

FIG 6–55.— Normal appearance and position of the ossification center for the medial epicondyle in a 7-year-old boy.

FIG 6–56.—Normal irregularities and pseudofractures of the ossification centers of the distal humerus in a 10-year-old girl. Note the lack of bilateral symmetry of some of these defects.

FIG 6–57.—A persistent epiphysis of the capitellum in an adult. *Left* and *center*, plain film. *Right*, tomogram. (From Nuvemann M: Einseitig ausgebliebene Verschmelzung des capitulum humeri: Eine seltene Manifestation der sogenannten persistierenden apophyse. *ROFO* 1982; 137:340. Used by permission.)

FIG 6–58.—Bilateral cleft epiphyses for the medial epicondyle in a 15-year-old boy. The left elbow was immobilized for 2 weeks on the assumption that the cleft represented a fracture. (Ref: Harrison RB, Keats TE: Epiphyseal clefts. *Skeletal Radiol* 1980; 5:23.)

FIG 6–59.—**A,** apparent displacement of the ossification center for the capitellum due to poor positioning of the forearm. **B,** proper position shows normal relationships.

FIG 6–60.—Marked asymmetry of ossification of the centers for the trochlea in an adolescent girl.

FIG 6–61.—Asymmetric development of the epiphyses for the capitellum in a 12-year-old boy. Such normal asymmetries in architecture and rate of growth are particularly common in the elbow and should not be misconstrued as evidence of trauma.

FIG 6–62.—A, simulated fracture of the ossification center of the medial epicondyle in a 14-year-old boy, produced by the superimposed radiolucent shadow of the growth plate between the ossification center and the bony side wall of the humerus (←). Note also the unusual appearance of the trochlea resulting from filming in a slight degree of flexion (↔). **B,** note the radiolucency of the growth plate of the trochlea in lateral projection.

FIG 6–63.— Normal irregularities in ossification of the capitellum, which should not be mistaken for fracture.

FIG 6–64.— Several simulated fractures of the ossification centers of the distal humerus in an 11-year-old boy. Such irregularities of ossification are common.

FIG 6–65.— Normal asymmetry in development of ossification centers. Note absence of the ossification center for the lateral epicondyle in **B** in an 11-year-old girl. (Ref: Silberstein MJ, et al: Some vagaries of the lateral epicondyle. *J Bone Joint Surg* 1982; 64A:444)

FIG 6–66.—Incomplete union of ossification centers for the epicondyles in a 44-year-old woman.

FIG 6–67.—Incomplete union of the ossification centers of the epicondyles in a 54-year-old woman.

FIG 6–68.—Examples of failure of union of ossification centers in adults.

FIG 6–70.—Projection of the middle eminence of the lower articular surface of the humerus.

FIG 6–69.—Patella cubiti, a sesamoid bone in the triceps tendon. (Ref: Kattan KR, Babcock DS: Bilateral patella cubiti. *Skeletal Radiol* 1979; 4:249.)

FIG 6–71.—Small bilateral ossicles related to the articular surface of the humerus. These may represent separate ossification centers for the middle eminence. Arthrograms indicate that they are enclosed in a lucent cartilage envelope. (Courtesy of Dr. Peter W. Cockshott.)

FIG 6–72.—Two examples of paratrochlear bones at the lateral humeral condyle. (Ref: Schwartz GS: Bilateral antecubital ossicles (fabella cubiti) and other accessory bones of the elbow. *Radiology* 1957; 69:730.)

FIG 6–73.—Probable bone island in the proximal portion of the ulna.

FIG 6–74.—Spur-like shadows, probably representing the edge of the capitellum in an 11-year-old boy.

FIG 6–75.—The posterior fat pad may be seen in some normal individuals with the elbow in extension. *Left,* partial flexion. *Right,* extension.

FIG 6–76.—**A,** simulated fracture through the epiphysis of the trochlea, produced by angulation of the beam. **B,** comparison view of the opposite elbow in true lateral projection shows similar lucency without simulated fracture.

FIG 6–77.—Another example of how the epiphysis of the trochlea may be mistaken for a fracture in the lateral projection.

FIG 6–78.—Normal asymmetry of development of the olecranon apophyses. Note irregular ossification in **B.**

FIG 6–79.—A separate nucleus of ossification for the olecranon process, not a fracture. (Ref: Silberstein MJ: Some vagaries of the olecranon. *J Bone Joint Surg* 1981; 63A:722.)

FIG 6–80.—Other examples of separate apical nuclei of ossification for the olecranon process.

FIG 6–81.—Bilaterally symmetric separate nuclei of ossification for the olecranon process in a 13-year-old boy.

FIG 6–82.—A, normal appearance of the uniting olecranon ossification center in an adolescent. **B,** incomplete union of the ossification center of the olecranon process—not a fracture—in an adult.

FIG 6–83.—Persistent unfused apophyses of the olecranon in a middle-aged man.

FIG 6–84.—Simulated fracture of the ulna produced by trabeculations in the shaft (←) and a small excrescence in the cortex just below the location of the distal end of the unossified apophysis (⟵).

FIG 6–85.—Unusual development of the olecranon in a single individual. **A,** ossicle. **B,** fossa.

FIG 6–86.—Residual irregularity of the olecranon after closure of the apophysis in a 19-year-old man.

FIG 6–87.—Normal foramina for nutrient vessels of the proximal ulna.

FIG 6–88.—Cancellous bone of the proximal end of the ulnae, simulating destructive lesions in a 49-year-old man.

FIG 6–89.—Cleft epiphysis of the radial head. (Ref: Harrison RB, Keats TE: Epiphyseal clefts. *Skeletal Radiol* 1980; 5:23.)

FIG 6–90.—Notches on the lateral aspects of the radial metaphyses in a 6-year-old girl. These are filled in by further growth and disappear as the child matures (see Fig 6–91).

FIG 6–91.—This patient illustrates the mechanism by which the notches seen in Figure 6–90 are obliterated. In **A** the fossa is being filled in by a separate center. In **B** the fossa is being filled in by overgrowth of the epiphysis of the radial head. This is the same mechanism seen for completion of growth of the tibial tubercle. These variants of growth may be mistaken for traumatic events. (Courtesy of Dr. Anne C. Brower.) (Ref: McCarthy SM, Ogden JA: Radiology of postnatal skeletal development: VI. Elbow joint, proximal radius and ulna. *Skeletal Radiol* 1982; 9:17.)

FIG 6–92.—Small cleft in the radial metaphysis in a 16-year-old girl, which should not be mistaken for a fracture (see Fig 6–112).

FIG 6–93.—Small cleft that might be mistaken for fracture in the lateral aspect of the proximal radial metaphysis. There was no history of trauma.

FIG 6–95.—Ossification center at the tip of the coronoid process of the ulna (os cubiti anterius) in an adolescent (see Figs 6–96 to 6–99). (Ref: Kohler A, Zimmer EA: *Borderlands of the Normal and Early Pathologic in Skeletal Roentgenology,* ed 3. New York, Grune & Stratton, 1968, p 132.)

FIG 6–94.— A small spur arising from the radial head.

FIG 6–96.—Accessory ossicle at the tip of the coronoid process.

FIG 6–97.—Accessory ossification centers for the tip of the coronoid process, which could be mistaken for a fracture.

FIG 6–98.—Persistent ossification center of the coronoid process of the ulna, which simulates a fracture.

FIG 6–99.—Partially fused ossicle at tip of the coronoid process of the ulna.

FIG 6–100.—Tendinous calcification at the coronoid process (←) in the origins of the flexor digitorum sublimis and at the insertion of the triceps tendon (↤). These should not be mistaken for traumatic sequelae.

FIG 6–101.—Examples of fossae in the ulna that represent the insertion point of the annular ligament. These should not be confused with a pathologic process. (Ref: Schoneich R: Tuberositas radii varietat "Bandgruber." *ROFO* 1988; 149:675.)

FIG 6–102.—Oblique radiolucent clefts in proximal radial metaphysis in a young child. These oblique clefts are a common finding adjacent to the epiphyseal lines in young children and should not be mistaken for metaphyseal fractures (see Fig 6–289). (Ref: Silberstein MJ, et al: Some vagaries of the radial head and neck. *J Bone Joint Surg* 1982; 64A:1153.)

FIG 6–103.—The radial tuberosity presents as a radiolucency and might be mistaken in both projections for an area of bone destruction.

FIG 6–104.—A radial tuberosity in a 4-year-old boy, simulating a focal destructive lesion only in the lateral projection.

FIG 6–105.—The interosseous ridges of the radius and ulna often cast shadows, which may be mistaken for periostitis.

FIG 6–106.—Physiologic "periostitis" of the newborn in a 2½-month-old infant. This is not seen before the age of 1 month and is symmetric in distribution, although not necessarily concentric, and may be seen in only one view. (Ref: Shopfner CE: Periosteal bone growth in normal infants: A preliminary report. *AJR* 1966; 97:154.)

FIG 6–108.—Normal undulations of the contour of the radii of the newborn. These disappear with increasing age.

FIG 6–107.—The nutrient channel of the radius.

FIG 6–109.—Cortical tunneling of the distal ulna may be seen in infants and older children and is of no clinical significance. (Ref: Weiss C: Normal roentgen variant: Cortical tunneling of the distal ulna. *Radiology* 1980; 136:294.)

FIG 6–110.—Small developmental metaphyseal spurs of the distal radius in a healthy 1-year-old girl.

FIG 6–111.—Normal metaphyseal irregularities of the radius in a 14-year-old boy. These changes were no longer present 1 year later. This alteration is probably similar to that illustrated in Figures 6–13, 6–52, 7–101, 7–110, 7–111, and 7–218.

FIG 6–112.—Small irregularities of the metaphysis in a 10-year-old girl (see Fig 6–92).

FIG 6–113.—Two examples of thin flanges of bone simulating periostitis of the distal radius.

FIG 6–114.—Examples of cortical irregularities at insertion of interosseous membrane simulating periostitis.

FIG 6–115.—Developmental fossa in distal ulna.

FIG 6–116.—Short ulna with a deep articulation with the radius, which resembles an erosive lesion. (Ref: Gelberman RH, et al: Ulnar variance in Kienböck's disease. *J Bone Joint Surg* 1975; 57A:674.)

FIG 6–117.—Unusually long ulnae, which may be mistaken for a dislocation of the distal radioulnar joint if the bilateral symmetry is not noted.

FIG 6–118.—*Left,* misdiagnosis of dislocation of the distal radio-ulnar joint by filming with wrist slightly rotated. *Right,* true lateral projection shows normal relationships.

FIG 6–119.—Normal spur-like projections of the epiphysis at the epiphyseal line, simulating avulsion injuries (see Fig 6–8). (Ref: Keats TE, Harrison RB: The epiphyseal spur. *Skeletal Radiol* 1980; 5:175.)

FIG 6–120.—Epiphyseal spurs on medial and lateral aspects of the distal radius.

FIG 6–121.—Residual epiphyseal spur after closure of the epiphyseal plate in a 20-year-old man.

FIG 6–122.—Closed epiphyseal spur mistaken for an avulsion fracture.

FIG 6–123.—Remnants of the epiphyseal line simulating a fracture in an 18-year-old man.

FIG 6–124.—Remnants of the epiphyseal line in a 20-year-old man.

FIG 6–125.—Small spicules in the epiphyseal cartilage of the ulna in a healthy 11-year-old girl. This is a normal finding of no significance.

FIG 6–126.—Spicules in the epiphyseal cartilage of the ulna in a 13-year-old boy.

FIG 6–127.—Closing distal radial epiphyseal line simulating a fracture. This situation prevails when the ulnar aspect of the distal radial epiphysis is thin, and the remnant of the epiphyseal line may be confused with an incomplete fracture. (From Teates CD: Distal radial growth plate remnant simulating fracture. *AJR* 1970; 110:578. Used by permission.)

FIG 6–128.—Simulated fracture of the radial epiphysis produced by superimposed projection of the epiphyseal plate at different levels.

FIG 6–129.—Cleft distal radial epiphysis seen only in the oblique projection. Any epiphysis or apophysis may develop from multiple centers (see Figs 6–130, 6–131, 7–123, 7–283, and 7–537). (Ref: Harrison RB, Keats TE: Epiphyseal clefts. *Skeletal Radiol* 1980; 5:23.)

FIG 6–130.—Examples of cleft distal ulnar epiphyses.

FIG 6–131.—Separate ossification centers for the radial styloid process, which may persist into adult life and be mistaken for fracture.

FIG 6–132.—Accessory ossicle of the end of the ulnar styloid, which should not be mistaken for a fracture.

FIG 6–133.—Accessory ossicles at the ulnar styloid, which articulate with the styloid process.

FIG 6–134.—Unusual length and configuration of the ulnar styloid processes.

FIG 6–135.—Not all styloid ossicles are developmental in origin; some may be of traumatic origin. *Left,* fracture of the ulnar styloid at age 16. *Right,* at age 26 the fracture fragment has evolved into an ossicle.

FIG 6–136.—Unusually long ulnar styloid process, which articulates with the triangular bone.

FIG 6–137.—Ring shadow on the ulnar styloid. This lesion is similar to other entities seen elsewhere in the wrist and hands that are probably fibrous in nature. They do not appear to be of clinical significance (see Figs 6–216 and 6–243).

FIG 6–138.—The vacuum phenomenon in the wrist joint.

1. Epitrapezium
2. Calcification (bursa, flexor carpi radialis)
3. Paratrapezium (petrapezium)
4. Trapezium secundarium
5. Trapezoides secundarium
6. Os styloideum
7. Ossiculum Gruberi
8. Capitatum secundarium
9. Os hamuli proprium
10. Os vesalianum
11. Os ulnare externum (calcified bursa or tendon)
12. Os radiale externum
13. Fissure of traumatic origin
14. Persisting ossification center of the radial styloid process
15. Intercalary bone between the navicular and the radius (paranavicular)
16. Os carpi centrale
17. Hypolunatum
18. Epilunatum
19. Accessory bone between the lunate and the triangular bone
20. Epipyramis
21. So-called "os triangulare"
22. Persisting center of the ulnar styloid
23. Small ossicle at the level of the radioulnar joint
25. Avulsion from the triangular bone; no accessory ossicle
26. Tendon or bursal calcification
27. Calcification of the pisiform

FIG 6–139.—The accessory ossicles of the hand (after Kohler). The sesamoid bones are indicated by *shaded circles*. (Ref: Kohler A, Zimmer EA: *Borderlands of the Normal and Early Pathologic in Skeletal Roentgenology,* ed 3. New York, Grune & Stratton, 1968.)

FIG 6–140.—Accessory ossicle at the radial styloid process, representing a persistent ossification center.

FIG 6–141.—The os styloideum. This ossicle lies between the capitate and the base of the second and third metacarpals. It produces a small immovable protuberance on the dorsum of the hand and may give rise to symptoms. (Refs: Bassöe E, Bassöe H: The styloid bone and carpe bossu disease. *AJR* 1955; 74:886; and Conway WE, et al: The carpal boss: An overview of radiographic evaluation. *Radiology* 1985; 156:29.)

FIG 6–142.—Two additional examples of the os styloideum.

FIG 6–143.—The os epilunatum.

FIG 6–144.—The os epitriquetrum (os epipyramis). This ossicle is located on the dorsal and radial edge of the triangular bone and varies in size. (Ref: Kohler A, Zimmer EA: *Borderlands of the Normal and Early Pathologic in Skeletal Roentgenology,* ed 3. New York, Grune & Stratton, 1968, p 111.)

FIG 6–145.—The os triangulare.

FIG 6–146.—Bilateral os triangulare. Some osseous elements in this area may represent old avulsions of the styloid process. This is not true in this illustration, which is of a normal variation. (Ref: Kohler A, Zimmer EA: *Borderlands of the Normal and Early Pathologic in Skeletal Roentgenology*, ed 3. New York, Grune & Stratton, 1968, p 112.)

FIG 6–147.—Accessory bones between the lunate and triangular bones, probably a variant of the os triangulare.

FIG 6–148.—The os hamuli proprium.

FIG 6–149.—Examples of the os vesalianum.

FIG 6–150.—Accessory centers of ossification for the tuberosity of the navicular.

FIG 6–151.—Calcified nodules in the flexor carpi radialis tendon.

FIG 6–152.—The os carpi centrale.

FIG 6–153.—The os paratrapezium.

FIG 6–154.—Two examples of the trapezium secundarium.

FIG 6–155.—The trapezium secundarium.

FIG 6–156.—Normal ossification centers do not always develop symmetrically, as evidenced in this 23-month-old child.

FIG 6–158.—Bipartite lunate in a young child.

FIG 6–157.—Accelerated bone age associated with excessive obesity. This 2-year-old boy has a bone age approximately three times his chronologic age. (Ref: Caffey J: *Pediatric X-Ray Diagnosis,* ed 7. Chicago, Year Book Medical Publishers, 1978, p 1137.)

FIG 6–159.—Bilateral hypoplastic lunates discovered as incidental findings after fracture of right wrist.

FIG 6–160.—Small os epilunatum.

FIG 6–161.—Two examples of asymptomatic and clinically unimportant bone islands in the capitate (←).
There is also a bone island in the lunate in the first example (↔).

FIG 6–162.—Vascular foramina in the capitate bone (←). A similar foramen is seen in the lunate (⧺).

FIG 6–163.—The vascular foramen of the lunate (←). A bone island is present in the navicular (⟻).

FIG 6–164.—Bone island in the lunate in a 14-year-old boy.

FIG 6–165.—Lucent cleft in the capitate, simulating a fracture.

FIG 6–166.—Deep fossa in the radial side of the capitate. The os carpi centrale may develop in this fossa (see Fig 6–152).

FIG 6–167.—The os carpi centrale present bilaterally in a child.

FIG 6–168.—A large os carpi centrale in an adult. (Ref.: Gercovich EO, Greenspan A: Case report 598. *Skeletal Radiol* 1990; 19:143.)

FIG 6–169.—The joint between the capitate and hamate may be poorly visualized in normal individuals and should not be mistaken for the changes of an inflammatory arthritis.

FIG 6–170.—*Left*, apparent loss of the joint space between the capitate and hamate due to inability of the patient to flatten the hand. Note similar overlap of navicular and lunate. *Right*, improved positioning shows normal relationships.

FIG 6–171.—*Top left*, poorly positioned PA view mistaken for fracture of the capitate due to overlap of the shadows of the capitate and hamate. *Top right*, correct positioning shows no fracture. *Bottom*, off-lateral projection of wrist shows simulated fracture of the posterior aspect of the capitate.

FIG 6–172.—Congenital fusion of the capitate and hamate. Carpal fusions may occur as isolated anomalies or be associated with congenital malformation syndromes. The isolated fusions usually involve bones of the same row, such as triquetrum-lunate, capitate-hamate, or trapezium-trapezoid, while syndrome-related fusions often go across rows, i.e., trapezium-scaphoid. (Ref: Poznanski AJ: *The Hand in Radiologic Diagnosis,* ed 2. Philadelphia, WB Saunders, 1984, p 201.)

FIG 6–173.—The os styloideum (see Figs 6–141 and 6–142).

FIG 6–174.—Bilateral congenital fusions of the capitate, hamate, and multangular bones.

FIG 6–175.—Variable relationships of capitate to lunate, depending on degree of flexion or extension of the hand.

FIG 6–176.—Congenital fusion of the lunate and triangular bones.

FIG 6–177.—Developmental cleft in the lateral aspect of the hamate.

FIG 6–178.—Elongated unciform process of the hamate, the origin of the flexor digiti quanti muscle (←). Note also the cyst-like shadow produced by the base of the unciform process (↤).

FIG 6–179.—Elongated unciform process of the hamate misdiagnosed as a fracture (←). The cleft of the base of the fifth metacarpal is normal (↤) (see Fig 6–230).

FIG 6–180.—The hamulus of the hamate in lateral projection. This should not be mistaken for a trapezium secundarium.

FIG 6–181.—Two examples of the os hamuli proprium. The unciform process of the hamate may ossify independently and give the impression of an accessory bone or a fracture. (Ref: Kohler A, Zimmer EA: *Borderlands of the Normal and Early Pathologic in Skeletal Roentgenology,* ed 3. New York, Grune & Stratton, 1968, p 95.)

FIG 6–182.—The os hamuli proprium. **A,** normal wrist. **B,** wrist with separate unciform process. Note absence of ring shadow. **C,** the os hamuli proprium seen in carpal tunnel projection. Rarely the hook of the hamate may be congenitally absent. (Ref: Seeger LL, et al: Case report 464: Bilateral congenital absence of the hook of the hamate. *Skeletal Radiol* 1988; 17:85.)

FIG 6–183.—Bilateral os hamuli proprium. Note absence of ring shadows in the hamates.

FIG 6–184.—Hypoplasia of the lesser multangular in a 13-year-old boy.

FIG 6–185.—The carpal tunnel projection may produce an end-on view of the fifth metacarpal superimposed on the carpal bones. This may produce a ring-like radiolucency that should not be mistaken for a pathologic process. (Ref: Fodor T, et al: Carpal tunnel ring artifact. *AJR* 1985; 144:765.)

FIG 6–186.—Irregularity of the radial aspect of the greater multangular, simulating a fracture.

FIG 6–187.—The os paratrapezium.

FIG 6–188.—Ring lesion in the greater multangular bone. These lesions are fibrous in nature and are seen elsewhere in the hand and wrist. They are apparently of no clinical significance (see Figs 6–216 and 6–243).

FIG 6–189.—Unilateral development of the navicular from multiple foci in an 11-year-old boy.

FIG 6–190.—*Left,* accessory ossification center for the navicular in a 10-year-old boy. *Right,* 5 months later showing partial incorporation of the center.

FIG 6–191.—Congenital fusion of the navicular and greater multangular. Such fusions are not uncommon and usually are of no significance. (Ref: O'Rahilly R: Survey of carpal and tarsal anomalies. *J Bone Joint Surg* 1953: 35A:626.)

FIG 6–192.—Two views of a bipartite navicular bone (←). Note the joint space. which is visible in both projections (⇔).

FIG 6–193.—Bilateral bipartite navicular bones. (Ref: Waugh RL, Sullivan RF: Anomalies of the carpus with particular reference to the bipartite scaphoid (navicular). *J Bone Joint Surg* 1950; 32A:682.)

FIG 6–194.—Bilateral bipartite navicular bone with aseptic necrosis of the proximal portion on the right.

FIG 6–195.—Partial division of the navicular bone, simulating a fracture. These clefts are best seen on the ulnar border (**A** and **B**) but may be seen on the radial border as well (**C**). (Ref: Kohler A, Zimmer EA: *Borderlands of the Normal and Early Pathologic in Skeletal Roentgenology,* ed 3. New York, Grune & Stratton, 1968, p 100.)

FIG 6–196.—Incomplete cleft simulating a fracture in the navicular in a 10-year-old girl.

FIG 6–197.—Simulated fracture of the navicular due to Mach effect of underlying radial styloid.

FIG 6–198.—A, simulated fracture of the navicular due to trabecular pattern. B, navicular view shows no fracture.

FIG 6–199.—Simulated fracture of the navicular due to trabecular pattern. *Left,* PA view. *Right,* magnification view.

FIG 6–200.—Trabecular pattern simulating fracture of the navicular.

FIG 6–201.—*Left,* simulated fracture of the navicular due to trabeculation. *Right,* navicular view shows no fracture but defines the trabecular nature of the pseudofracture.

FIG 6–202.—Developmental cleft on the radial border of the navicular.

FIG 6–203.—Simulated fracture of the navicular due to notch on lateral margin.

FIG 6–204.—Bone island in the navicular.

FIG 6–205.—Simulated cysts of the navicular produced by trabecular pattern. Navicular views showed no abnormality.

FIG 6–206.—Rotary dislocation of the navicular may be simulated by faulty positioning of the wrist at the time of filming. **A,** note position of the ulnar styloid, indicating rotation of the wrist. The foreshortened configuration of the navicular is similar to the appearance of rotary dislocation. **B,** correct positioning of the wrist. Navicular assumes a normal configuration. (Ref: Hudson TM, et al: Isolated rotatory subluxation of the carpal navicular. *AJR* 1976; 126:601.)

FIG 6–207.—A, simulated rotary dislocation of the navicular produced by filming in radial deviation of the wrist. B, normal appearance of navicular with ulnar deviation.

FIG 6–208.—Voluntary bilateral painless subluxation of the naviculars in a 27-year-old man. A–D, both wrists at rest. E–H, both wrists with navicular subluxated at will.

FIG 6–209.—The interval between the navicular and the lunate is not always a reliable indication of rotary dislocation of the navicular, since its width is dependent on the position of the thumb. Note change in interval between **A** and **B.**

FIG 6–210.—**A,** the navicular-lunate interval in normal individuals may be quite wide and is not an indication of traumatic dissociation in itself. **B,** film made in ulnar deviation shows normal appearance of the navicular and decrease in the navicular-lunate interval.

FIG 6–211.—Wide navicular lunate intervals in a 14-year-old boy. This appearance and that of Figure 6–210 seem to be related to underdevelopment of the lunate (in Fig 6–210) or underdevelopment of the proximal end of the navicular (in this case).

FIG 6–212.—Accessory ossification center for the tubercle of the navicular in a 10-year-old girl (→). Note also accessory ossification center at the distal end of the first metacarpal (↠).

FIG 6–213.—Accessory ossification center for the tubercle of the navicular, which failed to unite.

FIG 6–214.—Three examples of congenital fusion of the lunate and triangular bones. This is a relatively common site of fusion. In childhood, the fissure between the incompletely fused bones should not be mistaken for fracture **(B).** (Refs: Carlson DH: Coalition of the carpal bones. *Skeletal Radiol* 1981; 7:125; and Resnik CS, et al: Incomplete carpal coalition. *AJR* 1986; 147:301.)

FIG 6–215.—Incomplete coalition of the lunate and triangular bones.

FIG 6–216.—Ring lesions in the triangular bone. These lesions are probably fibrous in nature and are seen elsewhere in the hand and wrist. They are apparently of no clinical significance and should be distinguished from traumatic cyst due to occupational trauma (see Figs 6–188 and 6–243).

FIG 6–217.—Normal irregularity of the pisiform in an 11-year-old boy. This irregularity is seen only in the lateral projection.

FIG 6–218.—Developmental irregularity of the pisiform in an 11-year-old boy, simulating a fracture.

FIG 6–219.—Bilateral irregularities in development of the pisiforms in a 12-year-old boy.

FIG 6–220.—Variations in the pisiform bone. **A,** normal, but very large pisiform bone. **B,** bipartite pisiform bones.

FIG 6–221.—Bipartite pisiform bone.

FIG 6–222.—Exostosis-like process on the pisiform bone, a variation in development.

FIG 6–223.—Congenital fusion of the triangular and pisiform bones.

FIG 6–224.—Two examples of accessory ossification centers at the bases of the metacarpals in 3-year-old (**A**) and 4-year-old (**B**) children. This finding is usually of no significance but may be seen in greater incidence in children with skeletal age lag. (Ref: Snodgrasse RM, et al: The association between anomalous ossification centers in the hand skeleton, nutritional status and rate of skeletal maturation in children 5–14 years of age. *AJR* 1955; 74:1037.)

FIG 6–225.—Accessory ossification center at distal end of the first metacarpal (→) and at the base of the second metacarpal (→) in a 13-year-old boy.

FIG 6–226.—Remnants of closed secondary ossification centers in a 13-year-old boy.

FIG 6–227.—The clefts at the ulnar side of the base of the fifth metacarpal are particularly prone to misinterpretation as fracture.

FIG 6–228.—Clefts at the bases of the metacarpals may simulate fractures.

FIG 6–229.—Fossa at the base of the fifth metacarpal may suggest abnormality.

FIG 6–230.—Normal shadows at the bases of the metacarpals that may be mistaken for fractures, due to overlapping shadows between the third and fourth metacarpals (→); note also the normal fossa at the base of the fifth metacarpal (⇀).

FIG 6–231.—The fifth metacarpal may be broader than the others and may simulate abnormality.

FIG 6–232.—Bulges in the cortices at the bases of the fourth and fifth metacarpals.

FIG 6–233.—Overlapping shadows of bases of second and third metacarpals that simulate fracture.

FIG 6–234.—Normal lucency in the base of the second metacarpal simulating a cyst-like lesion.

FIG 6–235.—Another example of lesion shown in Fig 6–234.

FIG 6–236.—Ossicle between the bases of the second and third metacarpals.

FIG 6–237.—Simulated fractures of the bases of the fourth and fifth metacarpals.

FIG 6–238.—Accessory ossification center at the distal end of the first metacarpal, simulating a fracture.

FIG 6–239.—Two examples of accessory ossification centers at the distal end of the first metacarpal with spur at its medial margin. The epiphyseal spur is a normal variation (see Figs 6–8 and 6–119).

FIG 6–240.—Closing accessory ossification center at the distal end of the first metacarpal in a 14-year-old boy.

FIG 6–241.—Spurring of the margins of ossification centers for the heads of the metacarpals in a 13-year-old boy. These spurs are transient events in the development of the epiphysis and are additional examples of the epiphyseal spur. (Ref: Keats TE, Harrison RB: The epiphyseal spur. *Skeletal Radiol* 1980; 5:175.)

FIG 6–242.—Prominent developmental spur-like protuberances at the radial sides of the distal metaphyses of the metacarpals.

FIG 6–243.—Ring lesions in the heads of the metacarpals. These are probably fibrous in nature and are apparently of no clinical significance (see Figs 6–188 and 6–216).

FIG 6–244.—Normal exaggeration of the pitlike depression in the head of the fifth metacarpal (←). This does not represent an erosion. The more usual appearance is seen in the head of the fourth metacarpal in **B** (⊬).

FIG 6–245.—Developmental spur-like projection at the radial side of the base of the second metacarpal.

FIG 6–246.—Attempted formation of an accessory metacarpal, seen best in **B,** arising from the greater multangular.

FIG 6–247.—Duplication anomaly of the first metacarpal (←) with an intervening articulation (⇐).

FIG 6–248.—Normal relationships between the base of the first metacarpal and greater multangular. This relationship is at times mistaken for a subluxation. **A,** abduction of the thumb. **B,** adduction of the thumb. (Ref: Lasserre C, et al: Osteoarthritis of the trapeziometacarpal joint. *J Bone Joint Surg* 1949; 31B:534.)

FIG 6–249.—Two examples of the trapezium secundarium (see Fig 6–154).

FIG 6–250.—Unusual configuration of the dorsal aspect of the distal end of the first metacarpal.

FIG 6–251.—Short fourth metacarpals with positive metacarpal sign as a familial trait in a normal individual. Note the short middle phalanges of the fifth fingers, also a familial trait.

FIG 6–252.—The metacarpal sign. A tangent drawn through the distal ends of the fourth and fifth metacarpals normally does not intersect the head of the third metacarpal. **A,** normal. **B,** borderline. **C,** positive. A positive metacarpal sign is seen in some forms of gonadal dysgenesis but may also occur as a normal variant; its usefulness is therefore limited. (Ref: Bloom RA: The metacarpal sign. *Br J Radiol* 1970; 43:133.)

FIG 6–253.—Examples of stenosis of the medullary cavities of the metacarpals, a finding of no clinical significance.

FIG 6–254.—Normal palmar directed position of the head of the fifth metacarpal, not to be mistaken for displacement by trauma.

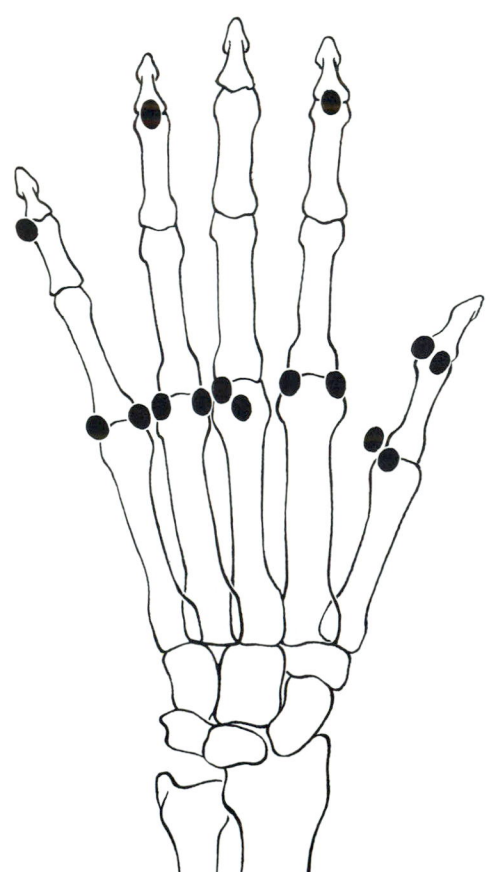

FIG 6–255.—Diagram of all the recognized sesamoid bones of the hand (after Degen).

FIG 6–256.—Sesamoid bone at the distal interphalangeal joint of the thumb.

FIG 6–257.—Unusual sesamoid in dorsal aspect of the distal interphalangeal joint of the thumb.

FIG 6–258.—Sesamoid bones at each metacarpal head in frontal (**A**) and oblique (**B**) projections.

FIG 6–259.—Solitary sesamoid bone at head of fourth metacarpal.

FIG 6–260.—Solitary sesamoids at the heads of the second metacarpals.

FIG 6–261.—Ossicle at the base of the proximal phalanx of the index finger, possibly a sesamoid.

FIG 6–262.—*Left,* supernumerary digits in the distal phalanges of an otherwise healthy 10-month-old child. *Right,* same patient at 19 years of age showing closing of the accessory centers of ossification. (Courtesy of Dr. N. Warn Courtney.)

FIG 6–263.—A, cleft epiphysis of proximal phalanx of the thumb seen in the oblique projection. **B,** cleft is not visible in frontal projection. (Ref: Harrison RB, Keats TE: Epiphyseal clefts. *Skeletal Radiol* 1980; 5:23.)

FIG 6–264.—Accessory centers of ossification of the epiphyses of the proximal phalanges, simulating avulsion injuries.

FIG 6–265.—Mach effect of metaphysis superimposing on epiphysis, suggesting a fracture.

FIG 6–266.—Attempt to form an accessory ossification center at the head of the proximal phalanx of the fourth finger in an 11-year-old boy. This might be mistaken for a fracture.

FIG 6–267.—Attempt to form an accessory ossification center at the distal end of the proximal phalanx of the thumb in a 10-year-old boy (→). Note similar process at the end of the metacarpal (⇸).

FIG 6–268.—Normal lucent fissures in the epiphyses in a 14-year-old boy, which may be mistaken for fractures.

474   *The Upper Extremity—The Fingers*

FIG 6–269.—Developmental cleft in the middle phalanges. *Left*, 9-year-old. *Right*, 10-year-old.

FIG 6–270.—Two examples of a small spur-like excrescence in the cortex of the proximal phalanx of the thumb, which probably represents the insertion of the extensor pollicis brevis tendon.

FIG 6–271.—*Left* and *center*, small incidentally found excresence at the base of the proximal phalanx of the fourth finger. *Right*, normal tuberosities of the bases of the phalanges, not to be mistaken for torus fractures.

FIG 6–272.—Small notches in the bases of the proximal phalanges should not be mistaken for the erosions of inflammatory arthritis, which should involve the heads of the metacarpals initially. (Ref: Stelling CB, et al: Irregularities at the base of the proximal phalanges. *AJR* 1982; 138:695.)

FIG 6–273.—Bilateral small spur-like projections from the bases of the proximal phalanges in a 20-year-old healthy woman.

FIG 6–274.—Normal ridges and projections of the proximal phalanx due to tendon sheath attachments, which may simulate periostitis or calcifying hematoma.

FIG 6–275.—Abortive attempt to form a triphalangeal thumb. There were no associated anomalies in this patient.

FIG 6–276.—Three examples of triphalangeal thumbs. (Ref: Theander G, Carstam N: Triphalangism and pseudotriphalangism of the thumb in children. *Acta Radiol [Diagn]* 1979; 20:223.)

FIG 6–277.—Normal irregularities of the palmar aspects of the first and second phalanges of the index finger.

FIG 6–278.—Exaggeration of normal irregularity of the head of the proximal phalanx of the third finger, not an exostosis.

FIG 6–279.—Osteosclerosis of the middle phalanx of the fifth finger.

FIG 6–280.—Bone island in the head of the proximal phalanx of the index finger.

FIG 6–281.—Nutrient foramina at the heads of the proximal phalanges. *Left*, 2-year-old child. *Right*, adult.

FIG 6–282.—Short middle phalanges of the fifth fingers are a finding associated with malformation syndromes, but may also be a normal familial trait as in this 18-year-old woman. (Ref: Greulich WW: A comparison of the dysplastic middle phalanx of the fifth finger in mentally normal Caucasians, Mongoloids and Negroes with that of individuals of the same racial groups who have Down's syndrome. *AJR* 1973; 118:259.)

FIG 6–283.—Anomalous development of the first metacarpals and the middle phalanges in a healthy 3-year-old child, representing a familial trait.

FIG 6–284.—*Left,* ivory epiphyses in the hands of children may occur as isolated events without clinical significance. This is more common in children with retarded maturation. (Refs: Kuhns LR, et al: Ivory epiphyses of the hands. *Radiology* 1973; 109:643; and Van der Laan JG, Thijn CJ: Ivory and dense epiphyses of the hand. *Skeletal Radiol* 1986; 15:117.)

FIG 6–285.—*Right,* normal relationships of the middle and distal phalanges of the thumb in a 9-year-old boy. Note wedged configuration of the epiphysis at the base of the distal phalanx.

FIG 6–286.—Speckled densities in the medullary cavities of the phalanges of both hands in a 58-year-old woman, probably representing prominent trabeculae in osteoporotic bone.

FIG 6–287.—Unusual clinodactyly of the fifth finger in an otherwise normal 14-year-old boy.

FIG 6–288.—Unusually large epiphysis of the base of the thumb.

FIG 6–289.—Horizontal fissure adjacent to the epiphyseal plate of the distal phalanx of the thumb in a 9-year-old child, not to be mistaken for a fracture (see Fig 6–102).

FIG 6–290.—Normal configurations of the terminal phalanges, which should not be mistaken for the effects of trauma.

FIG 6–291.—A and **B,** fossa in the base of the distal phalanx of the thumb may simulate a destructive lesion. **C,** lateral projection shows only the fossa. **D–F,** similar appearance is seen on the opposite side.

FIG 6–292.—Attempted bifid distal phalanx.

FIG 6–293.—Soft tissue laceration simulating fracture of the ungual tuft.

FIG 6–294.—Familial broad thumbs. Short, broad, distal phalanges of the thumbs are often seen in malformation syndromes but may also occur as normal familial traits.

FIG 6–295.—Sclerosis of the terminal phalanges is seen in the collagen diseases but may also occur in normal individuals, usually in females over the age of 40 years. (Ref: Goodman N: The significance of terminal phalangeal osteosclerosis. *Radiology* 1967; 89:709.) The sclerosis begins early in adult life and regresses with old age. (Ref: Fischer E: Akroostiosklerose der Finger, eine Normale Geschlects und Altersabbangige Endostale Reaktion. *ROFO* 1982; 137:384.)

FIG 6–296.—Bilateral terminal phalangeal sclerosis with varied degrees of involvement in a 60-year-old woman.

FIG 6–297.—Persistence of terminal phalangeal sclerosis in an 80-year-old woman.

FIG 6–298.—Terminal phalangeal sclerosis of a single digit.

FIG 6–299.—Soft-tissue calcification of the distal phalanges of the fingers, a finding of no clinical significance that may result from mechanical injury. (From Fischer E: Weichteilverkalkungen am Rand der uberositas phalangis distalis der Finger. *ROFO* 1983; 139:150–157. Used by permission.)

Chapter 7

The Lower Extremity

FIG 7–1.—This 2-year-old infant has Perthes disease on his left side. However, the defect in the head of the right hip is a developmental variant, not incipient osteochondrosis. **A,** hips in neutral position. **B,** hips in abduction. (Ref: Katz JF: "Abortive" Legg-Calvé-Perthes disease or developmental variation in epiphysiogenesis of upper femur. *J Mount Sinai Hosp NY* 1965; 32:651.)

FIG 7–2.—Normal irregular mineralization of the ossification center of one femoral head. This appearance in a single center in a young infant does not necessarily indicate disease. (Ref: Caffey J: *Pediatric X-Ray Diagnosis,* ed 8. Chicago, Year Book Medical Publishers, 1985, p 787.)

FIG 7–3.—Normal stippled appearance of one ossification center in a 10-month-old infant. These centers evolve to normal contour with further growth. (Ref: Lemperg R, et al: Asymmetry of the epiphyseal nucleus in the femoral head in stable and unstable hip joints. *Pediatr Radiol* 1973; 1:191.)

FIG 7–4.—Two examples of normal developmental irregularity of the femoral heads in children without hip symptoms. **A,** 3-year-old boy. **B,** 4½-year-old boy.

FIG 7–5.—Double ossification centers for the capital femoral epiphysis. This is a normal variant, not an indication of disease.

FIG 7–6.—Cleft of the proximal femoral epiphysis in a 3-year-old girl (see Figs 6–129, 7–123, and 7–283).

FIG 7–7.—Normal asymmetry in size of the ossification centers of the femoral heads may be seen normally and is not necessarily indicative of congenital dislocation of the femoral head.

FIG 7–8.—The femoral notch in two 9-year-old children. This defect is probably cartilaginous since it does not communicate with the joint on arthrography. It may be seen as early as 4 years and disappears gradually over the course of months or years. (Ref: Ozonoff MB, Ziter FMH Jr: The femoral head notch. *Skeletal Radiol* 1987; 16:19.)

FIG 7–9.—Two examples of the normal irregularity of the acetabular roofs in young children. This appearance is normal between the ages of 7 and 12 years.

FIG 7–10.—Apparent radiolucency of the femoral head in 5-year-old boy (→) produced by superimposition of the normal irregularities of the acetabulum at this age (↦) (see Fig 7–9).

FIG 7–11.—Normal intrapelvic protrusion of the acetabula. This is a normal phase of development between 4 and 12 years of age.

FIG 7–12.—The fossa at the entry point of the acetabular nutrient vessels may simulate a destructive lesion of the femoral head.

FIG 7–13.—**A,** unusually large bilateral fovea capitis, which may be mistaken for osteochondritis dissecans. **B,** tomogram of right hip.

FIG 7–14.—The same entity shown in Figure 7–13 in a 20-year-old man.

FIG 7–15.—Large fovea capitis in a 26-year-old man as in Figures 7–13 and 7–14.

FIG 7–16.—Simulated fracture or aseptic necrosis of the femoral head produced by the fovea capitis. **A,** plain film. **B,** laminagram. No fracture seen.

FIG 7–17.—Simulated destructive lesions of the femoral heads produced by superimposition of the acetabular bone on the femoral head. **A,** hips in neutral position. **B,** hips in abduction.

FIG 7–18.—The shadow of the posterior acetabular margin superimposed on the femoral head may simulate the density of aseptic necrosis.

FIG 7–19.—The lucent interval between the anterior (→) and posterior lips of the acetabulum (↠) may simulate a lucent lesion of the femoral head (⇥).

FIG 7–20.—Ossification centers for the acetabulum, which may simulate fractures, in a 14-year-old boy (see Figs 4–70 to 4–76).

FIG 7–21.—Ununited secondary ossification centers (os acetabuli marginalis superior) in a young adult (see Fig 4–82).

FIG 7–22.—The "vacuum" phenomenon in normal hips in a 6-month-old child. The *upper arrow* indicates an accessory ossification center for the transverse process of L-5.

FIG 7–23.—"Vacuum" phenomenon in the hips of an adult. Note how the radiolucency in **A** resembles a fracture line.

FIG 7–24.—Two examples of the unreliability of Shenton's line after the newborn period. **A,** 5-month-old infant. **B,** 1-year-old child. Note particularly the asymmetry of the lines in **A.**

FIG 7–25.—Apparent bulging of the hip "capsule," suggesting synovitis or hemarthrosis, may be produced by filming the hip in abduction and external rotation, as in this 6-year-old boy (→). Note normal fat lines on opposite side(↠). (Ref: Brown I: A study of the "capsular" shadow in disorders of the hip in children. *J Bone Joint Surg* 1975; 57B:175.)

FIG 7–26.—Plump femoral heads in a 22-month-old infant. (Courtesy of Dr. Clement Fauré.)

FIG 7–27.—Unusual configuration of the femoral heads in a 26-year-old man.

FIG 7–28.—In using the line drawn along the femoral necks for the detection of slipped capital femoral epiphysis, there is great normal variability in the amount of femoral head that is intersected. This is illustrated in these two adolescent boys.

FIG 7–29.—Normal irregularities of the metaphyseal bone at the epiphyseal line in early childhood. **A,** 4-year-old girl. **B,** 5-year-old boy.

FIG 7–30.—Normal double contour effect of cortex of superior aspect of the femoral neck in a 4-year-old boy. This is a common appearance in children of this age.

FIG 7–31.—The upper femoral notch (←) in a 13-year-old boy. This is probably the same lesion seen in the humeral neck (Fig 6–7) and other metaphyseal sites (Figs 6–52, 6–111, 7–100, 7–102, 7–110, and 7–218). The lesion disappears with growth and is of no significance. Note also the poor definition of the upper margin of the femoral neck (←), also a normal appearance at this age. (Ref: Ozonoff MB, Ziter FMH Jr: The upper femoral notch. *Skeletal Radiol* 1985; 14:198.)

FIG 7–32.—Two additional examples of the upper femoral notch.

FIG 7–33.—Normal irregularities and lucencies in the femoral necks of an 11-year-old boy.

FIG 7–34.—Normal lucencies in the femoral necks in a 16-year-old boy.

FIG 7–35.—Normal lucencies in the necks of the femora (Ward's triangle) formed by the angle of the trabeculae in the neck of the femur.

FIG 7–36.—Bilateral localized trabecular radiolucencies in the femoral necks of a healthy 53-year-old woman.

FIG 7–37.—*Top left*, normal triangular radiolucencies in the femoral necks produced by the heavy trabeculations in the center of the femoral neck and the overlap of the femoral head medially. *Top right*, this appearance may be asymmetric in its presentation. *Bottom left and right*, similar radiolucencies may be seen in the frog-leg projection.

FIG 7–38.—Relative radiolucencies in the femoral necks of an 85-year-old man produced by the large trabeculations of the femoral neck inferior and medial to the edge of the greater trochanter.

FIG 7–39.—Radiolucencies produced by overlap of the greater trochanter and the heavy trabeculation of the femoral neck in a 51-year-old man.

FIG 7–40.—Typical juvenile benign cortical defects are occasionally seen in the femoral neck and are of no clinical significance. **A,** 7-year-old boy. **B,** three years later, the lesion is slightly larger.

FIG 7–41.—Examples of ring-like radiolucencies of the femoral necks with sclerotic borders. These are common lesions that are apparently of no clinical significance. There is evidence to suggest that they represent a subcortical pit formed by herniation of synovium through the cortical bone. (Ref: Pitt MJ, et al: Herniation pit of the femoral neck. *AJR* 1982; 138:1115.)

FIG 7–42.—**A** and **B,** bilateral herniation pits in a 25-year-old man. **C,** CT demonstration.

FIG 7–43.—Examples of bony thickenings of the inferior aspect of the femoral necks, probably due to ossification of the inferior retinaculum of the synovial capsule. **A** and **B,** 34-year-old woman. **C,** 25-year-old woman. (**A** and **B** courtesy of Dr. Clement Fauré.) (Ref: Fauré C, et al: L'éperon pectineo-fovéal du col fémoral. *J Radiol* 1983; 64:505.)

FIG 7–44.—Localized reinforcement of major trabeculae in a 75-year-old osteoporotic woman that might be mistaken for insufficiency fracture.

FIG 7–45.—**A,** normal area of radiolucency of the femoral neck, which becomes more marked in osteoporotic individuals. **B,** this area of radiolucency simulates a pathologic fracture in patients with traumatic fracture of the femoral neck due to rotation of the head. After reduction, this appearance is no longer seen. (Ref: Pope TL Jr, et al: Pseudopathologic fracture of the femoral neck. *Skeletal Radiol* 1981; 7:129.)

FIG 7–46.— An additional example of a simulated destructive lesion following fracture of an osteoporotic femur.

FIG 7–47.—*Left*, simulated fracture of the femoral neck in a 68-year-old woman produced by hypertrophic lipping, best seen in the lateral projection (*right*).

FIG 7–48.—Two examples of skin folds simulating fractures of the femur.

FIG 7–49.—Prominent vertical striation of the bone of the femoral neck in a normal 12-year-old girl.

FIG 7–50.—Simulated periostitis of the femoral neck produced by overlapping shadow of the greater trochanter.

FIG 7–51.—Normal irregularity of the ossification centers of the greater and lesser trochanters in a 3-year-old girl.

FIG 7–52.—Normal irregularities of ossification of the greater trochanter in a 12-year-old boy.

FIG 7–53.—Normal irregularity of the trochanteric apophyseal line in a 7-year-old boy.

FIG 7–54.—Ossification variant of the greater trochanter in a 15-year-old boy, simulating a fracture.

FIG 7–55.—Simulated cyst of the femoral neck produced in abduction by the shadow of the greater trochanter.

FIG 7–56.—Normal osteosclerosis of the premature. This sclerosis is due to the proportionally thicker cortical bone and incomplete development of the medullary cavities. This appearance reverts to normal in the first weeks of life.

FIG 7–57.—Physiologic "periostitis" of the newborn. This is not seen before the age of 1 month and is symmetric in distribution, although not necessarily concentric, and may be seen in only one view. (Ref: Shopfner CE: Periosteal bone growth in normal infants: A preliminary report. *AJR* 1966; 97:154.)

FIG 7–58.—Additional examples of physiologic "periostitis" of the newborn seen in two 4-month-old infants. Incorporation is evident and is essentially completed by 6 months of age.

FIG 7–59.—Physiologic anterior bowing of the femurs in a 19-month-old, heavy girl. This is a self-limited phenomenon that disappears as the child matures. (Ref: Caffey J: *Pediatric X-Ray Diagnosis*, ed 8. Chicago, Year Book Medical Publishers, Chicago, 1985, p 812.)

FIG 7–60.—Combined anterior and lateral physiologic bowing of the tibias in a 12-month-old girl.

FIG 7–61.—The shadow of the fascia lata, which may simulate new bone formation.

FIG 7–62.—Muscle interleaved with fat may resemble a soft tissue mass, most commonly seen in women.

FIG 7–63.—Striking delineation of the muscles about the proximal femur in a young boy.

FIG 7–64.—Soft tissue companion shadow of the femur.

FIG 7–65.—Speckled trabeculation of the intertrochanteric area, which should not be mistaken for cartilaginous tumor matrix or bone infarction. These are reinforced trabeculae seen in osteoporotic bone (see Fig 7–66). (Ref: Kerr R, et al: Computerized tomography of proximal femoral trabecular patterns. *J Orthop Res* 1986; 4:45.)

FIG 7–66.—Development of the speckled pattern of the femur in a young woman immobilized after a stroke. **A,** baseline. **B,** 4 years later the bone has become osteopenic from disuse and speckles have appeared.

FIG 7–67.—The femoral linea aspera-pilaster complex for the insertion of the adductor and extensor muscles. (Ref: Pitt MJ: Radiology of the femoral linea aspera-pilaster complex: The track sign. *Radiology* 1982; 142:66.)

FIG 7–68.—*Left*, the pilaster complex misdiagnosed as a fracture of the femur *(arrows)*. *Right*, CT shows the cortical ridge *(arrow)* but no fracture.

FIG 7–69.—Bilateral linear intramedullary densities of the femurs in a 22-year-old woman. (Courtesy of Dr. J.C. Hoeffel.)

FIG 7–70.—Bilateral linear intramedullary densities of the femurs in a 67-year-old woman. These are seen more frequently in elderly women without known disease and are apparently of no clinical significance.

FIG 7–71.—*Left*, same entity as shown in Figures 7–69 and 7–70 in a 70-year-old woman.

FIG 7–72.—*Right*, unusual endocortical scalloping in a 70-year-old woman with no known disease, presumably representing a reflection of osteoporosis.

FIG 7–73.—Normal nutrient vascular channels of the femoral shaft.

FIG 7–74.—Nutrient foramen in a 7-year-old boy that, when added to the normal cortical thickening of the posterior aspect of the femur, was mistaken for an osteoid osteoma. *Left,* frontal projection. *Center,* lateral projection. *Right,* CT scan.

FIG 7–75.—The nutrient channel of the femur.

FIG 7–76.—Three examples of lucent fissures in the posterior cortex of the femur, which might be mistaken for fracture lines.

FIG 7–77.—Typical juvenile benign cortical defects. These lesions are very common in the distal femur and are of no clinical significance. (Refs: Caffey J: *Pediatric X-Ray Diagnosis,* ed 8. Chicago, Year Book Medical Publishers, 1985, p 446; and Ritschl P, et al: Fibrous metaphyseal defects: Determination of their origin and natural history using a radiomorphological study. *Skeletal Radiol* 1988; 17:8.)

FIG 7–79.—Healing juvenile benign cortical defect in a 17-year-old boy (←). Note mixed lucency and sclerosis. Note also longitudinal striations in the metaphysis, a common finding in young people. (⊬).

FIG 7–80.—Huge healed juvenile benign cortical defect in an 18-year-old woman.

FIG 7–81.—*Left*, very dense healed juvenile benign cortical defect in a 24-year-old woman.

FIG 7–82.—*Right*, prominent longitudinal striations of the bone in a normal 13-year-old girl.

FIG 7–83.—*Left*, "tug" lesion of the medial aspect of the distal femur in an adolescent, representing bone formation in the insertion of the adductor magnus muscle. (Ref: Barnes GR Jr, Gwinn JL: Distal irregularities of the femur simulating malignancy. *AJR* 1974; 122: 180.)

FIG 7–84.—*Right*, small "tug" lesion in an 11-year-old girl.

FIG 7–85.—Additional example of the "tug" lesion of the femur in an adult (→). Note also calcification in the medial collateral ligament (⇢) and an ossicle below of the same etiology (⧾).

FIG 7–87.— Bilateral "tug" lesions of the femur, probably secondary to pull of the vastus lateralis and medialis.

FIG 7–86.— Very large "tug" lesion of the medial femoral metaphysis resembling an osteochondroma.

FIG 7–88.— Bilateral cortical thickenings in a young man, probably related to muscle insertion, a common radiologic finding.

FIG 7–89.—A normal triangular area of radiolucency seen in the metaphysis of the distal femur in an osteoporotic individual (←). The density in the midportion is related to the linea aspera (⊬).

FIG 7–90.—Triangular radiolucency in an 11-year-old girl.

FIG 7–91.—Examples of transverse ("growth") lines of the distal femoral metaphyses. Although frequently associated with disease states, these lines are often seen in patients without contributory history.

FIG 7–92.—Detailed view of transverse lines of the distal femur in a younger child.

FIG 7–93.—Two examples of normal metaphyseal radiolucencies, an accompanying feature of the osteosclerosis of the newborn (see Fig 7–56). The new bone formed at the metaphysis is often more radiolucent, producing an appearance that might be mistaken for evidence of systemic disease. This finding is often the product of intrauterine stress.

FIG 7–94.—Dense zones of provisional calcification are often mistaken for the lines of heavy metal poisoning. These zones vary considerably in thickness in healthy children and in the same child at different ages. They tend to be proportionately thicker during the second to fifth years. (Ref: Caffey J: *Pediatric X-Ray Diagnosis,* ed 8. Chicago, Year Book Medical Publishers, 1985, p 481.)

FIG 7–95.—Additional examples of normal zones of provisional calcification. **A,** 14-month-old infant. **B,** 2-year-old infant.

FIG 7–96.—Simulated lesions of the femur produced by the edge of the growth plates in tunnel views in a 10-year-old boy.

FIG 7–97.—Incipient benign cortical defects in a 6-year-old boy. At this age, the defects are adjacent to the epiphyseal line, are ill defined, and do not have the sclerotic margins that are seen in older children (see Figs 7–77 and 7–78).

FIG 7–98.—Additional examples of early benign cortical defects in a 6-year-old boy.

FIG 7–99.—Nutrient foramen of the distal femur.

FIG 7–100.—Three examples of irregularity of the cortex of the anterior aspect of the femur, immediately above the epiphyseal line. This entity is seen in adolescence and is a transient event. **A,** 11-year-old boy. **B,** 13-year-old boy. **C,** 15-year-old boy (see Fig 7–101). (Ref: Keats TE: The distal anterior femoral metaphyseal defect: An anatomic variant that may simulate disease. *AJR* 1974; 121:101.)

FIG 7–101.—Irregular defect in the cortex of the medial posterior aspect of the distal femur is a common finding between the ages of 12 and 16 years. This is a fibrous lesion, which often demonstrates fine perpendicular spiculation of bone (**B**) and may be mistaken for a malignant bone tumor. It appears to be developmental in origin and disappears with advancing age. It seems to be similar in nature to other metaphyseal irregularities seen elsewhere in the body at the same age (see Figs 6–13, 6–52, 6–111, 7–100, 7–110, and 7–218). It is important to note that the metaphyseal irregularities in the medial posterior aspects of the distal end of the femur are cold on nuclear scanning, which would suggest that they are not avulsive in nature. (Refs: Brower AC, et al: The histologic nature of the cortical irregularity of the medial posterior distal femoral metaphysis in children. *Radiology* 1971; 99:389; and Burrows PE: The distal femoral defect: Technetium 99m pyrophosphate bone scan results. *J Can Assoc Radiol* 1982; 33:91.)

FIG 7–102.—Good detail of the architecture of the medial femoral cortical irregularity in a 15-year-old boy.

FIG 7–103.—Medial femoral cortical irregularity in a 13-year-old boy with large spur at the inferior margin of the lesion (←).

FIG 7–104.—Distal femoral cortical irregularities on both sides in a 10-year-old boy.

FIG 7–105.—Residuals of the irregularity of the cortex in the area of the medial femoral defects described in Figures 7–103 and 7–104. **A,** 17-year-old boy. **B,** 23-year-old man. **C,** 35-year-old man.

FIG 7–106.—**A,** typical benign cortical defect of the femur in a 12-year-old boy. **B,** follow-up film made 3 years later shows the typical medial cortical irregularity. This evolution lends weight to the concept of the similar nature of these two entities.

FIG 7–107.—The medial distal femoral cortical irregularity in a 13-year-old boy. Note the spiculations of bone *(arrow)* and the absence of cortex. The nuclear scan was normal.

FIG 7–108.—Coexistence of the medial posterior cortical defect (→) and a benign cortical defect (⊣⊢→).

FIG 7–109.—Two examples of normal irregularity in ossification of the posterior aspect of the distal femur in 2-year-old infants.

FIG 7–110.—Irregularity of the posterior aspect of the distal femur in adolescents is a common finding often mistaken for the new bone formation of a neoplasm. This lesion is apparently related to the medial cortical irregularity illustrated in Figure 7–101 and is of no clinical significance per se. It, too, is cold on nuclear scanning, which suggests that it is not an avulsive injury and is more likely to be a reflection of the same growth phenomena illustrated in Figures 6–13, 6–52, 6–111, 7–101, and 7–218. (Refs: Bufkin WJ: The avulsive cortical irregularity. *AJR* 1971; 112:487; and Burrows PE, et al: The distal femoral defect: Technetium 99m pyrophosphate bone scan results. *J Can Assoc Radiol* 1982; 33:91.)

FIG 7–111.—Large irregular posterior femoral defect in a 12-year-old girl proved by biopsy to be fibrous in nature.

FIG 7–112.—Well-defined posterior femoral defect in a 12-year-old girl.

FIG 7–113.—Residual posterior distal femoral defects in an 18-year-old girl, which can be seen in the frontal projection **(B)** as radiolucencies that might be mistaken for evidence of pathology.

FIG 7–114.—Residuals of the posterior femoral defect in a 30-year-old man.

FIG 7–115.—Four examples of cortical irregularities in the posterior cortex of the distal femur that have persisted into adult life, presumably the end product of the process shown in Figures 7–110 and 7–111. These defects are important only because they might be mistaken for significant lesions.

FIG 7–116.—Simulated lesions of the anterior aspect of the distal femur produced by rotation at the time of filming.

FIG 7–117.—Physiologic bowing and knock-knee. **A,** physiologic bowing in a 1½-year-old girl. **B,** physiologic knock-knee in a 3½-year-old girl. In normal development, there is a varoid phase to the age of 2 years and a valgoid phase between 2 and 12 years of age. These are normal physiologic events that correct spontaneously. (Refs: Holt JF, et al: Physiological bowing of the legs in young children. *JAMA* 1954; 154:390; and Shopfner CE, Coin CG: Genu varus and valgus in children. *Radiology* 1969; 92:723.)

FIG 7–118.—Physiologic bowing. Note the slight beaking of the medial tibial plateaus, the medial wedging of the ossification centers of the knees, and the thickening of the medial cortices of the tibias. These are all reflections of this physiologic state (see Fig 7–121, A).

FIG 7–119.—Physiologic knock-knees in a 3-year-old boy. Note lack of any architectural derangement.

FIG 7–120.—Evolution of physiologic bowing. **A,** age 18 months. **B,** 2 years of age, showing spontaneous correction. **C,** 4 years of age. The appearance is normal.

FIG 7–121.—**A,** 1-year-old girl with physiologic bowing. Note the "fragmentation" of the medial aspect of the tibial metaphysis (→). **B,** same patient at age 2. Note conversion to mild knock-knee deformity and resolution of the changes of physiologic bowing.

FIG 7–122.—Asymmetric development of the distal femoral epiphysis in a 7-year-old boy with no symptoms referable to the knee joints. (see Figs 6–129 and 7–123).

FIG 7–123.—Cleft distal femoral epiphysis seen only in the lateral projection. Any epiphysis or apophysis may develop from multiple centers (see Figs 6–129, 7–283, and 7–537).

FIG 7–124.—Normal irregularity of ossification of the medial femoral metaphyses in young children.

FIG 7–125.—Normal irregularities in ossification at the knees of young infants. (Ref: Caffey J, et al: Ossification of the distal femoral epiphysis. *J Bone Joint Surg* 1958; 40A:647.)

FIG 7–126.—Additional examples of normal irregularities of the distal femoral epiphyses in 1-year-old children.

FIG 7–127.—A, normal developmental lucency of the lateral aspects of the distal femoral epiphysis, simulating a destructive lesion in a 6-year-old boy. **B,** similar, but less marked, changes are present in the opposite limb.

FIG 7–128.—*Top,* normal developmental lucencies in the epiphyses and metaphyses of the distal femur in a 10-year-old boy.

FIG 7–129.—*Center,* developmental radiolucent stripes in the medial aspect of the distal femoral epiphysis, simulating fracture. **A,** 5-year-old boy. **B,** 7-year-old boy.

FIG 7–130.—*Bottom,* normal irregular contours of the distal femoral epiphyses in a 4-year-old girl.

FIG 7–131.—An excellent example of the normal irregularity of the distal femoral epiphyses in an 8-year-old girl that explains the misleading shadows seen in the frontal projections of the knees of children of this age.

FIG 7–132.—Normal irregularity of the lateral condyles of the femur in a 7-year-old boy. These irregularities are posteriorly located and are seen in the tunnel views of both knees (**B** and **C**) but not in the conventional anteroposterior projection (**A**). (Ref: Caffey J, et al: Ossification of the distal femoral epiphysis. *J Bone Joint Surg* 1958; 40A:647.)

FIG 7–133.—Medial and lateral femoral condylar irregularities seen in the tunnel views of both knees of a 10-year-old boy. These irregularities are often mistaken for evidence of osteochondrosis.

FIG 7–134.—Simulated osteochondrosis dissecans in a 6-year-old boy.

FIG 7–135.—Normal developmental irregularities of the condyles in a 12-year-old boy, not to be mistaken for osteochondrosis. (Ref: Caffey J: *Pediatric X-Ray Diagnosis,* ed 8. Chicago, Year Book Medical Publishers, 1985, p 443.)

FIG 7–136.—Simulated osteochondrosis dissecans in an 11-year-old boy. Note that the irregularities are not seen in the frontal projection *(top left)*, are well demonstrated in the tunnel projection *(top middle)*, and are seen posteriorly in the lateral projection *(top right)*. MR shows normal appearance of the articular cartilage *(bottom left and right)*.

FIG 7–137.—Normal irregularities in ossification of the lateral femoral condyle in an 8-year-old boy. **A,** frontal projection. **B,** oblique projection. **C,** lateral projection.

FIG 7–138.—Accessory ossification center of the distal femoral epiphysis seen in lateral projection.

FIG 7–139.—Spur-like configuration of the medial femoral epiphysis in a 12-year-old girl, not an epiphyseal osteochondroma. (Ref: Kohler A, Zimmer EA: *Borderlands of the Normal and Early Pathologic in Skeletal Roentgenology,* ed 3. New York, Grune & Stratton, 1968, p 415.)

FIG 7–140.—*The normal notch of the lateral condyle seen in the lateral projection (**A**) may reflect itself in the frontal plane (**B**) in a manner that suggests an abnormality.*

FIG 7–141.—Two additional examples of normal contour irregularities of the condyles seen in lateral projection. This contour alteration may be seen in the patellar view as well (see Fig 7–143).

FIG 7–142.—**A,** simulated lesion of the anterior surface of the femoral condyle produced by rotation. **B,** normal appearance in repeat examination.

FIG 7–143.—Normal contour alteration of the lateral condyle seen in tangential projection (see Fig 7–141).

FIG 7–144.—The grooves of the distal articular surface of the femur represent a normal variant, which should not be confused with osteochondrosis or fracture. (Ref: Harrison RB, et al: The grooves of the distal articular surface of the femur—a normal variant. *AJR* 1976; 126: 751.)

FIG 7–145.—The groove for the popliteal tendon shuld not be mistaken for a pathologic process.

FIG 7–146.—The grooves of the popliteal tendon seen in the tunnel view.

FIG 7–147.—An ossicle in the popliteal groove. (Cyamella sesamoid in the popliteal tendon.)

FIG 7–148.—A large cyamella with overgrowth of the superior margin of the popliteal groove.

FIG 7–149.—Bilateral cyamellae in shallow popliteal grooves.

FIG 7–150.—Normal areas of sclerosis of the intercondylar fossae in a 25-year-old man.

FIG 7–151.—Apparent ossification variant of the medial femoral condyle in a 13-year-old boy. **A,** AP projection shows faint radiolucency. **B,** lateral projection shows no abnormality. **C,** PA MR T1-weighted image shows signal alteration in area of interest. **D,** lateral MR shows a subchondral osseous defect. This entity bears a resemblance to the femoral head notch illustrated in Figure 7–8 and was not related to the patient's symptoms.

FIG 7–152.—Normal radiolucent anterior segment of the distal femoral epiphysis in a 12-year-old boy, due to the fact that less bone is traversed anteriorly than posteriorly.

FIG 7–153.—Normal radiolucency, simulating a cystic lesion.

FIG 7–154.—Triangular area of radiolucency, which may be confused with the defect of osteochondrosis dissecans. (Ref: Weisman JC: The medial femoral triangle of radiolucency simulating osteochondrosis dissecans. *AJR* 1947; 58:166)

FIG 7–155.—Stippled appearance of distal femur due to closing epiphyseal plate in a 13-year-old boy. This appearance should not be confused with chondroid matrix of a neoplasm.

FIG 7–156.—Two examples of the foramina for the nutrient vessels of the distal end of the femur.

FIG 7–157.— Variations in development of the fabella. **A,** double fabella. **B,** bifid fabella. **C,** irregular fabella.

FIG 7–158.— Fat pad between joint capsule and quadriceps tendon, which may be mistaken for a lipohemarthrosis. (Ref: Butt WP, et al: Radiology of the suprapatellar region. *Clin Radiol* 1983; 34:511.)

FIG 7–159.—The vacuum phenomenon in the knee joint.

FIG 7–160.—Simulated narrowing of the medial compartments of the knees in a 14-year-old girl. This misleading appearance is the result of the double contour of the medial tibial plateau. Measurements should be made from the articular surface of the distal femoral condyle to the most distal of the tibial articular margins *(arrows).* Measured in this fashion, the width of both compartments is equal. (Ref: Fife RS, et al: Relationship between arthroscopic evidence of cartilage damage and radiographic evidence of joint space narrowing in early osteoarthritis of the knee. *Arthritis Rheum* 1991; 34:377.)

FIG 7–161.—**A** and **B,** simulated medial compartment narrowing on standing film on the same basis as Figure 7–160. This problem can also be resolved by tunnel projection **(C),** which demonstrates equality of measurement of both compartments.

FIG 7–162.—Some normal individuals show true asymmetry in the height of the medial and lateral compartments. *Top left,* male aged 48 years. Standing films show asymptomatic symmetrical narrowing of medial compartments. *Top right,* the same individual 10 years later shows no change in compartment height, and MR examination at this time shows normal articular cartilage. These variations are probably related to known normal differences in thickness of articular cartilage in normal individuals. (Ref: Hall FM, Wyshak G: Thickness of articular cartilage in the normal knee. *J Bone Joint Surg* 1980; 62A:408.)

FIG 7–163.—Small excrescences on the articular surface of the femur.

FIG 7–164.—Normal irregularity of the growing patellae in a 7-year-old boy.

FIG 7–166.—Normal irregularity and clefts in the patella of a 6-year-old boy.

FIG 7–167.—Normal variation in development of the patella in an 8-year-old boy, simulating a fracture.

FIG 7–168.—Normal developmental irregularities of the patellae, seen in the tangential projection. **A,** 7-year-old. **B,** 15-year-old.

FIG 7–169.—Three examples of accessory ossification centers at the superior pole of the patella.

FIG 7–170.—**A** and **B,** irregular patellar ossification, misdiagnosed as fracture. **C,** simulated fracture lines in the normal patella of a 7-year-old boy. **D,** normal irregularity of the superior aspect of the patella in a 12-year-old boy, simulating osteochondrosis or fracture.

FIG 7–171.—Unusual patterns of ossification of the patella in a 6-year-old boy.

FIG 7-173.—Apparent fracture of the superior aspect of the patella in a 14-year-old boy due to a secondary ossification center at the superior pole. (Ref: Ogden JA: Radiology of postnatal skeletal development: X. Patella and tibial tuberosity. *Skeletal Radiol* 1984; 11:246.)

FIG 7-174.—Normal asymmetric development of accessory ossification centers in a 9-year-old. Note apparent fragmentation of the lower pole of the patella in **B.**

FIG 7–175.—Long secondary apophysis of the anterior and inferior aspects of the patella in an 11-year-old boy.

FIG 7–176.—Three examples of accessory ossification centers simulating fracture. **A,** 7-year-old boy. **B,** 8-year-old boy. **C,** 12-year-old boy.

FIG 7–177.—*Left,* accessory ossification center in an 8-year-old boy diagnosed as a fracture. *Right,* film made 1 month later with no treatment shows progressive closure of the secondary center.

FIG 7–178.—Variable patterns of ossification of the inferior pole of the patella.

FIG 7–179.— Accessory centers of ossification at the lower pole of the patella, which may be mistaken for fracture.

FIG 7–180.—**A,** the closing accessory center at the inferior pole of the patella was suspected of being a fracture, and a comparison view was made of the opposite knee **(B),** showing an even more misleading appearance.

FIG 7–181.—A, fusing accessory centers of ossification at the inferior pole of the patella. **B,** after fusion is complete. Patellae with large accessory centers of this type often tend to attain the elongate configuration illustrated in **B.** They may be associated with patella alta.

FIG 7–182.—Unfused accessory ossification center at the inferior pole of the patella in a 19-year-old man showing its closure over a 3-month period.

FIG 7–183.— Accessory patellar ossification center seen in tangential projection in a 12-year-old boy.

FIG 7–184.— Unusual spur-like configuration of the lateral aspect of the patella in a 20-year-old man.

FIG 7–185.— Bipartite patella, which may easily be mistaken for a fracture. Note the well-defined space between the major elements.

FIG 7–186.—An additional example of a bipartite patella, which is well demonstrated in tangential projection. The rounded contour of the patellar elements seen in this projection is useful in the differentiation from fracture.

FIG 7–187.—**A,** segmented patellae with two pieces on patient's right and three on the left. **B** and **C,** segmented patella with four pieces.

FIG 7–188.—A, unilateral bipartite patella. Note that the smaller element in bipartite patellae often does not accurately correspond in size with the adjacent fossa. **B,** unilateral bipartite patella (→) but with corresponding fossa on opposite side (↠). **C** and **D,** bipartite patella on the medial side. The majority of bipartite patellae are located on the lateral side. *(Continued.)*

FIG 7–188 (cont.).—E–G, a tripartite patella. Note rounded contours in tangential projection (see Fig 7–189).

FIG 7–189.—Fossa in lateral margin of patella (see Fig 7–188, B).

FIG 7–190.—A, the smaller element of a bipartite patella is usually smaller than the fossa in the major portion. However, occasionally it is larger than the fossa **(B).**

FIG 7–191.—Segmented patella showing poor definition of septae in the oblique projection *(right)*.

FIG 7–192.—Horizontal bifid patella, a rare type of segmentation. (Ref: Weinberg S: Horizontal bifid patella. *Skeletal Radiol* 1981; 7:223.)

FIG 7–193.—Accessory ossicle at medial aspect of patella.

FIG 7–194.—Lucent cleft in the anterior aspect of the patella seen only in the tangential projection.

FIG 7–195.—Patellar "teeth" due to spurring of the tendon interdigitations. (Ref: Greenspan A, et al: "Tooth" sign in patellar degenerative disease. *J Bone Joint Surg* 1977; 59A:483.)

FIG 7–196.—**A** and **B** show the dorsal patellar defect. These cortical lucencies are of no clinical significance and should not be confused with osteochondrosis dissecans of the patella. **C,** 1 year later. Note sclerosis of healing. **D,** 2 years later. Resolution is complete. (Ref: Haswell DM, et al: The dorsal defect of the patella. *Pediatr Radiol* 1976; 4:238.)

FIG 7–197.—Bilateral dorsal patellar defects in a 13-year-old girl.

FIG 7–198.—Dorsal patellar defects in a 12-year-old girl.

FIG 7–199.—Dorsal defects in an elderly male. These defects are seen more commonly in young people but occasionally persist into later life. *Top left*, frontal view. *Top right*, lateral view. *Bottom*, tangential views.

FIG 7–200.—Bilateral areas of density in the posterior surfaces of the patella in a 20-year-old woman.

FIG 7–201.—Simulated fracture of the upper pole of the patella produced by a small flange-like projection, best seen in lateral projection.

FIG 7–202.—The lucency of the upper pole of the patella seen in Figure 7–201 is nicely demonstrated in this 33-year-old man.

FIG 7–203.—Simulated stress fracture of the patella on the same basis as Figure 7–202. Note that no discontinuity is seen in the lateral projection *(top right)* or in the tomogram *(bottom)*.

FIG 7–204.—Unusual configurations of the lower poles of the patellae. **A** and **B**, 12-year-old boy. **C**, 14-year-old girl.

FIG 7–205.—Two examples of ossicles or sesamoid bones in the patellar tendon.

FIG 7–206.— A third tibial spine.

FIG 7–207.—An ossicle in the intercondylar notch.

FIG 7–208.—The third (←) and fourth (⊢) tibial condyles. (Ref: Kohler A, Zimmer EA: *Borderlands of the Normal and Early Pathologic in Skeletal Roentgenology,* ed 3. New York, Grune & Stratton, 1968, pp 440–441.)

FIG 7–209.—An ossicle at the fourth tubercle on the dorsal aspect of the proximal tibial surface. Note also marked concavity of the posterior aspect of the patella. (Ref: Kohler A, Zimmer EA: *Borderlands of the Normal and Early Pathologic in Skeletal Roentgenology,* ed 3. New York, Grune & Stratton, 1968, p 441.)

FIG 7–210.— Normal depressions in the anterior tibia of a 4-year-old. These depressions disappear with the development of the ossification center for the tibial tubercle.

FIG 7–211.—Normal variations in appearance of the apophysis of the tibial tubercle. None of these are necessarily indicative of Osgood-Schlatter disease.

FIG 7–212.—The edge of the proximal tibial epiphysis as seen in lateral projection may simulate a fracture.

FIG 7–213.—Three additional examples of normal variation in appearance of the ossification center of the tibial tubercle in adolescence.

FIG 7–214.—A separate, ununited ossification center for the tibial tubercle in a young adult. This should not be confused with a fracture.

FIG 7–215.—The unfused ossification centers for the tibial tubercle seen in the tangential view **(B).**

FIG 7–216.—Large tibial tubercle simulating an intra-articular loose body on tangential projection *(arrow).*

FIG 7–217.—Ring-like lesions in the proximal tibia are of no clinical significance. They are probably fibrous in nature. Similar lesions are seen in the pelvis (Fig 4–40), femur (Fig 7–35), and fibula (Fig 7–264).

FIG 7–218.—A, medial metaphyseal cortical irregularity of the tibia in an adolescent. This is a developmental phenomenon similar to that seen in the humerus (Figs 6–13 and 6–52), the radius (Fig 6–111), and the femur (Figs 7–100, 7–101, and 7–110). B, on follow-up, the irregularity was replaced by a typical benign cortical defect, suggesting the interrelationship of these lesions.

FIG 7–219.—Normal fossae at the medial tibial metaphysis should not be mistaken for erosions. In the elderly, they appear exaggerated because of spurring of the joint margin.

FIG 7–220.—Developmental notch on the medial aspect of the tibial plateau in a 15-year-old boy.

FIG 7–221.—Small spur at the medial tibial metaphysis, probably representing a "tug" lesion produced by the tibial collateral ligament.

FIG 7–222.—Developmental bulge of the medial tibial metaphysis.

FIG 7–223.—A, simulated fracture of the proximal tibia due to rotation at the time of filming. B, correct position shows no fracture.

FIG 7–224.—Accessory ossification center at the proximal end of the fibula.

FIG 7–225.—Accessory ossicle at the superior end of the fibula in a 44-year-old man.

FIG 7–226.—Normal lucency in the proximal fibular epiphysis in a 15-year-old girl (see Fig 6–19 for a similar finding in the humeral head.)

FIG 7–227.—Ununited accessory ossification center at the head of the fibula, simulating a fracture (←). Note also the bifid fabella (⟨⟩).

FIG 7–228.—Metaphyseal irregularity of the medial aspect of the fibular metaphysis in a 13-year-old boy. This represents the same kind of alteration seen in the metaphyses of other long bones at this age (see Figs 6–13, 6–52, 6–111, 7–100, 7–101, 7–110, and 7–218).

FIG 7–229.—Developmental flange-like expansion of the neck of the fibula in a 15-year-old boy (see Fig 7–232).

FIG 7–230.—Two examples of simulated discontinuity of the cortex of the fibula in lateral projection, which may be mistaken for fracture.

FIG 7–231.—Simulated cyst of the head of the fibula due to the large amount of cancellous bone present in this area.

FIG 7–232.—"Tug" lesions at the metaphysis of the proximal fibula due to the insertion of the soleus muscle, not to be mistaken for an osteochondroma.

FIG 7–233.—Example of marked "tug" lesions of the fibula in a 12-year-old long-distance swimmer. (Courtesy of Dr. John Farwaker.)

FIG 7–234.—The soleal line represents a "tug" lesion due to the origin of the soleus muscle. It should not be mistaken for periostitis. (Ref: Levine AH, et al: The soleal line: A cause of tibial pseudope-riostitis. *Radiology* 1976; 119:79.)

FIG 7–235.—"Tug" lesions at both ends of the soleus muscle, producing a fibular spur (←) and the soleal line (↔).

FIG 7–236.—The open apophysis for the tibial tubercle, which should not be mistaken for fracture.

FIG 7–237.—Simulated fracture of the tibia produced by overlapping of the fibula posteriorly *(arrow)* and trabeculations anteriorly.

FIG 7–238.—Radiolucency produced by the tibial tubercle en face.

FIG 7–239.—Three examples of pseudoperiostitis, simulated by the tibial tuberosity *(arrows)*. (Ref: Kohler A, Zimmer EA: *Borderlands of the Normal and Early Pathologic in Skeletal Roentgenology,* ed 3. New York, Grune & Stratton, 1968, p 442.)

FIG 7–240.—Laminated appearance of the tibial tubercle, not to be confused with periosteal new bone formation.

FIG 7–241.—Apparent fracture of the neck of the fibula produced by rotation and overlap of the open apophysis of the tibial tubercle.

FIG 7–242.—Thickening of the anterior cortex of the tibia, producing an unusual appearance in the frontal projection.

FIG 7–243.—A, simulated dislocation of the head of the fibula produced by filming in slight rotation. Note medial position of the patella. B, opposite side showing proper positioning and normal relationships.

FIG 7–244.—Short fibula.

FIG 7–245.—Physiologic bowing of the fibula in a 19-month-old child, which should not be mistaken for a plastic bowing fracture.

FIG 7–246.—Physiologic bowing of the fibulae in an 11-year-old boy.

FIG 7-247.—Normal posterior bowing of the fibulae in an adult.

FIG 7-248.—Spurious thickening of the lateral cortex of the tibia due to slight external rotation of the leg. The density is due to the fact that the anterior tibial crest comes progressively more into profile. (Ref: Caffey J: *Pediatric X-Ray Diagnosis,* ed 8. Chicago, Year Book Medical Publishers, 1985, p 455.)

FIG 7-249.—Normal cortical irregularities of the shafts of the fibulae. *Left,* frontal projection. *Right,* lateral projections.

The Lower Extremity—The Shafts of the Tibia and Fibula   **587**

FIG 7–250.—Localized bilateral symmetric undulations in the fibular cortex.

FIG 7–251.—**A,** notch-like lesion in distal fibula seen in the oblique projection. Note similarity to a like defect in the humerus (Fig 6–45). **B,** lesion not seen in the frontal projection.

FIG 7–252.—Normal irregularities of the cortices of the tibia and fibula due to ossification of the interosseous membrane.

FIG 7–253.—Simulated isolated periostitis of the tibia as in Figure 7–252.

FIG 7–254.—Localized ossification in the interosseous membrane.

FIG 7–255.—Two examples of juvenile benign cortical defects of the tibia. These lesions are common in the tibia and are of no clinical significance. (Ref: Caffey J: *Pediatric X-Ray Diagnosis*, ed 8. Chicago, Year Book Medical Publishers, 1985, p 446.)

FIG 7–256.—Two additional examples of benign cortical defects of the tibia.

FIG 7–257.—Two examples of healed juvenile benign cortical defects.

FIG 7–258.— Very dense healed benign cortical defects.

FIG 7–259.— Nutrient vascular channels of the fibula.

FIG 7–260.— Nutrient channels of the fibula mistaken for fracture.

FIG 7–262.—The nutrient channel of the tibia.

FIG 7–261.—Three examples of nutrient foramina of the fibula that might be mistaken for fractures.

FIG 7–263.—Normal bump in the medial cortex of the distal fibula of a 2-year-old child, which may simulate a torus fracture.

FIG 7–264.—Ring-like lesions of the distal fibula. These are probably similar in nature to those seen in the proximal end of the tibia (Fig 7–217) and are of no clinical significance.

FIG 7–265.—Tibial flange that might be mistaken for an avulsion fracture.

FIG 7–266.—Normal localized angulation of the distal epiphyseal plate of the tibia in an 11-year-old boy.

FIG 7–267.—The epiphyseal impression illustrated in Figure 7–266 should not be mistaken for a fracture in the lateral projection.

FIG 7–268.—Two examples of normal localized depressions in the metaphyses of the distal fibula in 11-year-old boys (←). The angulation of the distal tibial epiphysis is also seen in **B** (⊬). (Ref: Ogden JA, McCarthy SM: Radiology of postnatal skeletal development. VIII. Distal tibia and fibula. *Skeletal Radiol* 1983; 10:209.)

FIG 7–269.—Normal radiolucencies in the distal fibular metaphyses in a 10-year-old boy.

FIG 7–279.—Residuals of the epiphyseal line of the fibula in a 19-year-old.

FIG 7–280.—The fibular ossicle, a normal fibular accessory ossification center, in a 12-year-old boy. In **A,** it is seen at the lateral aspect of the fibular metaphysis. In **B,** there is a large ossicle at the lateral aspect of the epiphyseal line. These ossicles fuse after puberty and are often mistaken for fractures. A large os subfibulare is also present in **A** (⊹). (Ref: Caffey J: *Pediatric X-Ray Diagnosis,* ed 8. Chicago, Year Book Medical Publishers, 1985, p 459.)

FIG 7–281.—Another example of the fibular ossicle.

FIG 7–282.—Three examples of fibular ossicles, all misinterpreted and treated as fractures.

FIG 7–283.—Cleft distal tibial epiphysis seen only in the oblique projection. Such clefting may be seen in many locations in late childhood (see Figs 6–129, 6–130, 7–123, 7–284, and 7–537).

FIG 7–284.—Cleft tibial epiphysis on the lateral side in a 16-year-old boy (see Fig 7–283).

FIG 7–285.—Bilateral metaphyseal defects in a 4-year-old boy, probably related to the metaphyseal defects seen in older children (see Figs 6–52, 6–111, 7–100, 7–101, 7–110, and 7–218).

FIG 7–286.—Cleft distal fibular metaphyses in a 7-year-old boy.

FIG 7–287.—Normal localized radiolucency of the distal end of the fibula due to cancellous bone.

FIG 7–288.—Developmental fossae in the medial aspects of the distal fibulae.

FIG 7–289.—Simulated fractures of the posterior malleolus produced by Mach effect of overlap of the tibia and fibula.

FIG 7–290.—Irregularity of mineralization of the medial edge of the distal tibial epiphysis in an 8-year-old. This is similar to that seen in the distal femoral epiphysis (see Fig 7–125).

FIG 7–291.—Bilateral separate secondary ossification centers for the medial malleoli in an 8-year-old boy, which may be mistaken for fractures.

FIG 7–292.—Normal irregular ossification of the tip of the medial malleolus in adolescent children. In **C,** an ossicle is seen between the calcaneus and the lateral malleolus, which represents the os trochleae calcanei (⟊). (Ref: Ogden JA, McCarthy SM: Radiology of postnatal skeletal development: VIII. Distal tibia and fibula. *Skeletal Radiol* 1983; 10:209.)

FIG 7–293.—Bilateral multicentric ossification of the medial malleolus in a 9-year-old girl.

FIG 7–294.—**A,** medial malleolar ossicle simulating a fracture in frontal projection. **B,** oblique projection shows cortication of an ossicle.

FIG 7–295.—Closing accessory ossification center for the medial malleolus in an 8-year-old boy.

FIG 7–296.—A, developmental radiolucency in the medial malleolus in a 9-year-old boy secondary to the presence of a secondary ossification center. **B,** follow-up 4 months later shows closing of secondary ossification center.

FIG 7–297.—Persistent, irregular ossification of the medial malleolus in an adult.

FIG 7–298.—Large bilateral os subtibiale, accessory ossification centers that have persisted into adult life and are frequently mistaken for fractures.

FIG 7–299.—The os subtibiale. This is a rare accessory bone related to the posterior colliculus of the medial malleolus, as opposed to the more common os subtibiale, which is related to the anterior colliculus that forms the tip of the malleolus. (From Coral A: The radiology of skeletal elements in the subtibial region: Incidence and significance. *Skeletal Radiol* 1987; 16:298. Used by permission.)

FIG 7–300.—Unfused accessory ossification center of the distal tibia producing unusual appearance of the upper margin of the talus. **A,** frontal projection. **B,** oblique projection. **C,** tomogram.

FIG 7–301.—Bony flanges on medial aspect of medial malleolus, which should not be mistaken for avulsion injuries.

FIG 7–302.—Normal band of density in the articular surface of the posterior malleolus.

FIG 7–303.—Small fossa on the articular surface of the posterior malleolus of no clinical significance.

FIG 7–304.—Normal undulations of the cortex of the posterior malleolus.

FIG 7–305.—Irregular mineralization of the distal end of the lateral malleolus, which should not be mistaken for fracture.

FIG 7–306.—Secondary ossification center of the lateral aspect and distal end of the lateral malleolus in a 12-year-old girl.

FIG 7–307.—Large os subfibulare at the tip of the lateral malleolus with inset into the adjacent malleolus.

FIG 7–308.—Large os subfibulare. **A,** an 11-year-old boy. **B,** a 14-year-old boy. Ossicles in this location may be symptomatic in children. (Ref: Griffiths JD, Menelaus MB: Symptomatic ossicles of the lateral malleolus in children. *J Bone Joint Surg* 1987; 69B:317.)

FIG 7–309.—A, os subfibulare seen only in oblique projection. **B,** frontal projection.

FIG 7–310.—Simulated fracture of the tip of the lateral malleolus due to trabeculations. Note that the cortical margins are intact.

FIG 7–311.—Os subfibulare (→) with deep fossa in distal end of the fibula (↦).

FIG 7–312.—Large os subfibulare mistaken for a fracture. This ossicle can sometimes be differentiated from a fracture by mentally subtracting the ossicle from the fibula and determining whether the architecture of the fibula is correct without the additional osseous element.

FIG 7–313.—Two examples of the os subfibulare. **A,** multiple irregular fragments that have persisted into adult life in a 19-year-old man. **B,** large solitary, flat nucleus that might be confused with a fracture fragment, since the typical pointed end of the fibula has not been achieved.

FIG 7–314.—Incomplete fusion of the ossification center for the lateral malleolus in an adult, simulating a fracture.

FIG 7–315.—Scale-like secondary ossification centers that resemble fractures.

FIG 7–316.—Spur-like extension of the distal end of the lateral malleolus.

FIG 7–317.—The os talotibiale, an accessory ossicle.

FIG 7–318.—"Foramen" in the lateral malleolus detected as an incidental finding (see Fig 7–296).

FIG 7–319.—Stress views of a normal ankle demonstrate the degree of joint widening. This is subject to great variability and illustrates the need for comparison views of the opposite side.

FIG 7–320.—Pseudotalar tilt produced by improper positioning of the foot at the time of filming. (Ref: Bigongiari LR: Pseudotibiotalar slant: A positioning artifact. *Radiology* 1977; 122:669.)

FIG 7–321.—Accessory skeletal elements as seen on an anteroposterior radiograph of the ankle joint. (Ref: Kohler, A, Zimmer EA: *Borderlands of the Normal and Early Pathologic in Skeletal Roentgenology,* ed 3. New York, Grune & Stratton, 1968.)

1. Accompanying shadow on the internal malleolus (patella malleoli)
2. Intercalary bone (or sesamoid) between the internal malleolus and the talus
3. Os subtibiale
4. Talus accessorius
5. Os sustentaculi
6. Os tibiale externum
7. Os retinaculi
8. Intercalary bone (or sesamoid) between the external malleolus and the talus
9. Os subfibulare
10. Talus secundarius
11. Os trochleare calcanei
12. Os trigonum

FIG 7–322.— The accessory bones of the foot (after Kohler). (Ref: Kohler A, Zimmer EA: *Borderlands of the Normal and Early Pathologic in Skeletal Roentgenology,* ed 3. New York, Grune & Stratton, 1968.) The sesamoid bones are indicated by *shaded circles.* These ossicles are usually of no clinical significance, but their recognition is important in the differential diagnosis of fracture. (Ref: Zatzkin HR: Trauma of the foot. *Semin Roentgenol* 1970; 5:419.)

1. Os tibiale externum
2. Processus uncinatus
3. Os intercuneiforme
4. Pars peronea metatarsalia
5. Cuboides secundarium
6. Os peroneum
7. Os vesalianum
8. Os intermetatarseum
9. Os supratalare
10. Talus accessorius
11. Os sustentaculum
12. Os trigonum
13. Calcaneus secundarius
14. Os subcalcis
15. Os supranaviculare
16. Os talotibiale

FIG 7–323.—The os talocalcanei. (Ref: Kohler A, Zimmer EA: *Borderlands of the Normal and Early Pathologic in Skeletal Roentgenology,* ed 3. New York, Grune & Stratton, 1968, p 488.)

FIG 7–324.—The talus secundarius (←). Secondary ossification centers are seen at the medial malleolus (⇤).

FIG 7–325.—The talus accessorius.

FIG 7–326.—The os supratalare.

FIG 7–327.—Variable appearance of the os trigonum. The multicentric appearance in **A** might be mistaken for a fracture.

FIG 7–328.—A, the os trigonum may closely simulate a fracture of the posterior process of the talus. **B,** it also may require laminagraphy for resolution.

FIG 329.—A, the os trigonum in the oblique projection may not be evident as an isolated entity in the lateral projection **(B).**

FIG 7–330.—The os talotibiale.

FIG 7–331.—A multicentric os talotibiale.

FIG 7–332.—The os supratalare.

FIG 7–333.—Two examples of the os sustentaculum tali, seen in lateral projections, simulating a fracture of the articular surface of the calcaneus. (Ref: Kohler A, Zimmer EA: *Borderlands of the Normal and Early Pathologic in Skeletal Roentgenology,* ed 3. New York, Grune & Stratton, 1968, p 488.)

FIG 7–334.—Two accessory bones of the calcaneal tuberosity. **A,** the os subcalcus (←). An os supranaviculare is also present (╫). (Ref: Kohler A, Zimmer EA: *Borderlands of the Normal and Early Pathologic in Skeletal Roentgenology,* ed 3. New York, Grune & Stratton, 1968, p 486.) **B,** accessory bone arising from the tip of the trochlear process on the lateral wall of the calcaneus, seen in oblique projection. (Ref: Caffey J: *Pediatric X-ray Diagnosis,* ed 8. Chicago, Year Book Medical Publishers, 1985, p 468.)

FIG 7–335.—The calcaneus secundarius.

FIG 7–336.—An unnamed ossicle at the inferior aspect of the distal portion of the calcaneus.

FIG 7–337.—Two examples of the os supranaviculare. This ossicle is often confused with an avulsion fracture.

FIG 7–338.—Bilateral os supranaviculare.

FIG 7–339.—Large os supranaviculare.

FIG 7–340.—Huge os supranaviculare with articulations with both the talus and navicular.

FIG 7–341.—Large, bilateral os tibiale externum.

FIG 7–342.—Bipartite os tibiale externum.

FIG 7–343.—Partially fused os tibiale externum (accessory navicular).

FIG 7–344.—Virtually complete fusion of the os tibiale externum to the navicular bone (cornuate navicular).

FIG 7–345.—An unnamed ossicle adjacent to the navicular bone. Probably an ununited center of ossification.

FIG 346.—The os peroneum.

FIG 7–347.—Large, multicentric os peroneum.

FIG 7–348.—The os peroneum in frontal projection.

FIG 7–349.—Three examples of multicentric os peroneum.

FIG 7–350.—Unusual os peroneum.

FIG 7–351.—The os peroneum may be high in position and superimposed on the cuboid.

FIG 7–352.—Bipartite os peroneum simulating fracture.

FIG 7–353.—A large os peroneum that articulates with the cuboid.

FIG 7–354.—An os peroneum simulating partial coalition of the cuboid and calcaneus (←). Note the simulated fusion between the second cuneiform and third metatarsal (↞) (see Fig 7–442).

FIG 7–355.—Unnamed ossicle between the navicular and first cuneiform.

FIG 7–356.—Huge os vesalianum (see Fig 7–461).

FIG 7–357.—Huge os vesalianum fused to the base of the fifth metatarsal.

FIG 7–358.—Six examples of the variable appearance of the os intermetatarseum. Note the accessory ossicle at the distal end in **F.**

FIG 7–359.—The os trigonum, which should not be mistaken for fracture of the posterior process of the talus (see Fig 7–327).

FIG 7–360.—Huge posterior process of the talus.

FIG 7–361.—**A,** the os trigonum may be projected onto the talus and simulate a fracture. **B,** true lateral projection shows usual appearance of the os trigonum.

FIG 7–362.—An unusual os trigonum that articulates with the posterior process of the talus *(arrow)*.

FIG 7–363.—The os accessorium supracalcaneum seen prominently on the left and minimally on the right *(arrows)*. This ossicle is separate from the posterior process of the talus and articulates with the posterosuperior margin of the calcaneus. (From Milgrom C, et al: Open-quiz solution: Case report 341. *Skeletal Radiol* 1986; 15:150. Used by permission.)

FIG 7–364.—Two examples of normal saucer-like depressions on the superior aspect of the talus. (Ref: Resnick D: Talar ridges, osteophytes and beaks: A radiologic commentary. *Radiology* 1984; 151:329.)

FIG 7–365.—Os supratalare.

FIG 7–366.—Two examples of the talar beak illustrating its varied appearance. This structure is a developmental variant that should not be confused with hypertrophic spurring seen adjacent to the talonavicular joint.

FIG 7–367.—Two additional examples of the talar beak.

FIG 7–368.—Examples of very large talar beaks. Note in **B** that an accessory ossicle may develop at the distal end. (Ref: Keats TE: Hypertrophy of the talar beak. *Skeletal Radiol* 1979; 4:37.)

FIG 7–370.—Prominent trabecular pattern simulating fracture of the talus.

FIG 7–369.—Talar beak with two large articulating ossicles.

FIG 7–371.—Simulated fractures of the talus produced by prominent trabeculae.

FIG 7–372.—Simulated fracture of the talus produced by overlapping of the lateral malleolus and posterior process of the talus.

FIG 7–373.—Unusual width of the subtalar joint simulating talocalcaneal dislocation produced by poor positioning for the lateral projection. Note the foreshortening of the talus in the vertical plane.

FIG 7–374.—Simulated talocalcaneal coalition produced by improper positioning during filming. (Ref: Shaffer HA, Harrison RB: Tarsal pseudocoalition: A positional artifact. *J Can Assoc Radiol* 1980; 31:236.)

FIG 7–375.—The talus accessorius.

FIG 7–376.—Partially fused talus secundarius.

FIG 7–377.—Bilateral os sustentaculi. There are accessory bones lodged at the posterior end of the sustentaculum tali, slightly to its superior side. **A** and **B,** frontal projections. **C** and **D,** lateral projections. **E** and **F,** axial projections of the calcaneus. (Ref: March HC, London RI: The os sustentaculi. *AJR* 1956; 76:1114.) This anomaly may be incorporated in an accessory joint between the sustentaculum tali and the talus. (Ref: Bloom RA, et al: The assimilated os sustentaculi. *Skeletal Radiol* 1986; 15:455.)

FIG 7–378.—The fossa on the superior aspect of the talus in **A** (→) may produce apparent abnormalities in the oblique projections (**B** and **C**, ⇢).

FIG 7–379.—The nutrient foramen of the talus.

FIG 7–380.—A, deep fossa on the superior aspect of the talus in an adult producing apparent abnormalities in the frontal and oblique projections (**B** and **C**).

FIG 7–381.—Talus partitus, an unusual developmental anomaly in which the talus is partitioned. **A,** right ankle—plan film. **B** and **C,** tomograms—right ankle. **D,** similar but less marked appearance of the left talus (see Fig 7–363). (Ref: Schreiber A, et al: Talus partitus. *J Bone Joint Surg* 1985; 67B:430.) (Courtesy of Dr. L. W. Bassett.)

FIG 7–382.—Bilateral calcaneal hypoplasia in a 1½-year-old child.

FIG 7–383.—Variations in appearances of double ossification centers for the body of the calcaneus. This entity is seen in infants with bone dysplasias and occasionally in infants with no other obvious abnormality. **A,** a newborn with cleft center of calcaneus. **B,** a 2-year-old with two well-defined centers of ossification. **C–E,** fusing duplicate centers.

FIG 7–384.—Closing bilateral duplicate ossification centers of the calcaneus.

FIG 7–385.—Four examples of transient developmental calcaneal spurs in infants. This represents a variation in growth and disappears by 1 year of age. **A** and **B** are in the same child. (Refs: Robinson HM: Symmetrical reversed plantar calcaneal spurs in children. *Radiology* 1976; 119:187; and van Wiechen PJ: Reversed calcaneal spurs in children. *Skeletal Radiol* 1987; 16:17.)

FIG 7–386.—Four examples of simulated calcaneal cysts due to the normal arrangement of the trabecular pattern in this area. The presence of the nutrient channel within the cyst, as in **A,** is useful in identifying the area of radiolucency as a pseudocyst. This variant is confused with true cysts of the calcaneus. (Ref: Keats TE: The calcaneal nutrient canal. *Skeletal Radiol* 1979; 3:239.)

FIG 7–387.—The problem of distinguishing the pseudocyst (**A**) from a true cyst is most simply solved by using the axial projection of the calcaneus on which the pseudocyst will not be apparent (**B**).

FIG 7–388.— *Left,* accessory anomalous soleus muscle producing a soft tissue mass anterior to the Achilles tendon. *Right,* the opposite side is normal. (From Nidecker AC, et al: Accessory muscles of the lower calf. *Radiology* 1984; 151:47. Used by permission.) (Ref: Apple JS, et al: Accessory soleus muscle. Case report 376. *Skeletal Radiol* 1986; 15:398.)

FIG 7–389.—Normal variations in appearance of the growing calcaneus in adolescence. The irregularity of the calcaneal tuberosity before fusion of the secondary ossification center, as well as the density and fragmentation of the secondary ossification center, is a normal manifestation of growth.

FIG 7–390.—Simulation of fracture of the calcaneal tuberosity by the apophysis in the oblique projection of the foot. This is seen before the calcaneal apophysis is closed and is produced by projection of the caudal tip of the apophysis into the soft tissues, as illustrated in the oblique view **(A)**. This appearance is not always duplicated on the other foot **(B)**. (From Keats TE: Four normal anatomic variations of importance to radiologists. *AJR* 1957; 78:89. Used by permission.)

FIG 7–391.—Two more examples of the tip of the ossification center of the calcaneal tuberosity, seen in oblique projection.

FIG 7–392.—Appearance of the calcaneal apophyses in an adolescent. This projection may show centers of ossification that are not visible in the lateral projection.

FIG 7–393.—Simulated fractures of the calcaneus produced by the unfused secondary ossification center for the calcaneal tuberosity.

FIG 7–394.—Incomplete closure of the distal portion of the calcaneal apophysis in a 15-year-old boy.

FIG 7–395.—Failure of union of a portion of the calcaneal apophysis in an adult.

FIG 7–396.—A secondary ossification center at the tip of the trochlear process on the lateral wall of the calcaneus, seen well only in the oblique projection (←). The trochlear process may be so prominent, as in this case, as to suggest an exostosis (⇥). (Ref: Caffey J: *Pediatric X-Ray Diagnosis,* ed 8. Chicago, Year Book Medical Publishers, 1985, p 469.)

FIG 7–397.—Large trochlear processes of the calcaneus resembling an exostosis. (Ref: Kohler A, Zimmer EA: *Borderlands of the Normal and Early Pathologic in Skeletal Roentgenology,* ed 3. New York, Grune & Stratton, 1968, p 481.)

FIG 7–398.—The os subcalcis, not an avulsion fracture. (Ref: Kohler A, Zimmer EA: *Borderlands of the Normal and Early Pathologic in Skeletal Roentgenology,* ed 3. New York, Grune & Stratton, 1968, p 486.)

FIG 7–399.—Developmental fossae in the calcaneal tuberosity, seen in oblique projection.

FIG 7–400.—Developmental foramina in the calcaneal tuberosities, seen in oblique projection. This entity is probably related to the one in Figure 7–399.

FIG 7–401.—Nutrient channel of the calcaneus (→) and a fossa (→), which might be mistaken for an abnormality.

FIG 7–402.—Calcification in the plantar fascia in a healthy 24-year-old man, a finding not of clinical significance per se.

FIG 7–403.—The calcaneus secundarius should not be mistaken for a fracture of the anterior process of the calcaneus.

FIG 7–404.—Three examples of simulated fractures of the superior margin of the calcaneus produced by the sustentaculum tali.

FIG 7–405.—Simulated fracture of the calcaneus in lateral projection produced by overlapping shadow of the distal fibular epiphysis in an 8-year-old girl.

FIG 7–406.—Simulated fractures produced by the sustentaculum tali.

FIG 7–407.—Simulated fracture of the calcaneus produced by the sustentaculum tali. **A,** plain film. **B,** tomogram.

FIG 7–408.—Simulated cyst produced by the sustentaculum tali.

FIG 7–409.—An incomplete osseous bridge between the calcaneus and the cuboid.

FIG 7–410.—Prominent trabeculation in the calcaneus mistaken for a stress fracture. This is a rather common finding.

FIG 7–411.—Normal ossification of the navicular from duplicate irregular centers in a 6-year-old.

FIG 7–412.—Duplicate ossification centers of the navicular of different sizes.

FIG 7–413.—Irregular ossification of the tarsal navicular mistaken for Kohler's disease in a 5-year-old boy.

FIG 7–414.—Developmental irregularity of the medial aspect of the naviculars in a 12-year-old boy.

FIG 7–415.—Simulated cyst of the navicular produced by configuration of upper cortical margin.

FIG 7–416.—Normal ossification of the navicular from multiple centers in an 8-year-old boy. This appearance may be confused with osteochondrosis or a fracture.

FIG 7–417.—Incomplete fusion of duplicate ossification centers for the navicular in an 8-year-old boy, simulating fracture.

FIG 7–418.—Bilateral bipartite tarsal naviculars in an adult. Note the unusual configuration of the bone in the frontal projections. (Ref: Kohler A, Zimmer EA: *Borderlands of the Normal and Early Pathologic in Skeletal Roentgenology,* ed 3. New York, Grune & Stratton, 1968, p 495.)

FIG 7–419.—Bipartite navicular. **A,** frontal view. **B,** lateral view. **C,** frontal tomogram. Note similarity to findings in Figure 7–418.

FIG 7–420.—The os tibiale externum may be mistaken for a fracture (see Figs 7–341 to 7–344). This variant may occasionally be symptomatic. (Refs: Lawson JP, et al: The painful accessory navicular. *Skeletal Radiol* 1984; 12:250; and Grogan DP, et al: The painful accessory navicular: A clinical and histopathological study. *Foot Ankle* 1989; 10:164.)

FIG 7–421.—Huge os tibiale externum.

FIG 7–423.—Bilateral, partial fusion of the os tibiale externum to the navicular. The *arrows* point to the remnants of the line of fusion.

FIG 7–422.—Fusion of an os tibiale externum to the navicular.

FIG 7–425.—Unusual bilateral os tibiale externum.

FIG 7–424.—Configuration of the naviculars, suggesting complete incorporation of the os tibiale externum (cornuate navicular).

FIG 7–426.—The os tibiale externum in frontal *(left)* and lateral *(right)* projection.

FIG 7–427.—The os tibiale externum in lateral projection simulating a fracture of the cuboid.

FIG 7–428.—**A** and **B,** the os tibiale externum originally diagnosed as a fracture because of its presence on one side only. **C,** tomogram confirming nonfracture.

FIG 7–429.—Partial fusion of the os tibiale externum mistaken for a fracture.

FIG 7–431.—Normal irregularity of the joint margins of the navicular and cuboid in oblique projection. This entity should not be mistaken for a manifestation of arthritis.

FIG 7–432.—Unusual configuration of superior aspect of the navicular.

FIG 7–433.—Spur-like configuration of the navicular.

FIG 7–434.—*Top*, large navicular with spur-like extension posteriorly *(arrow)*. *Bottom*, a similar appearance is seen on the opposite side.

FIG 7–435.—Normal irregular ossification of the tarsal bones of the right foot in a 4-year-old child (**A–C**). Note bipartite ossification of calcaneus and talus as well as the irregularity of the cuneiforms. **D,** right foot at age 6. Note residual irregularities in the posterior aspect of the talus. **E,** left foot at age 6. Note some persistence of the bifid calcaneus.

FIG 7-436.—Irregular ossification of the cuneiforms in a 4-year-old boy.

FIG 7-437.—Irregular ossification of the first cuneiforms in a 6-year-old boy.

FIG 7-438.—Bilateral accessory ossification centers at the tip of the first cuneiform in a 9-year-old boy.

FIG 7–439.—Bilateral bipartite first cuneiforms in a 6-year-old. (Ref: Kohler A, Zimmer EA: *Borderlands of the Normal and Early Pathologic in Skeletal Roentgenology,* ed 3. New York, Grune & Stratton, 1968, p 511.)

FIG 7–440.—Confusing appearance at base of first metatarsal, simulating fracture in a 15-year-old boy, produced by overlapping shadows of the first cuneiform and the epiphysis of the base of the first metatarsal. The epiphyseal line at the base of the metatarsal is seen in **C** and demonstrated by tomography in **D.**

FIG 7–441.—Simulated fractures produced by overlapping shadows of the cuneiforms.

FIG 7–442.—The overlapping relationships illustrated in Figure 7–441 are better defined in the adult.

FIG 7–443.—*Left,* simulated fusion between the base of the third metatarsal and the lateral cuneiform. *Right,* situation clarified by filming in greater obliquity.

FIG 7–444.—Normal spacing between the first and second cuneiforms (←), not to be confused with traumatic alteration. The groove on the medial surface is also normal (⊬) (see Fig 7–445).

FIG 7–445.—Contour alterations of the second cuneiform mistaken for a fracture.

FIG 7–446.—Groove for the tibialis anterior tendon, not an erosion.

FIG 7–447.—Normal radiolucencies seen in and between the cuneiforms.

FIG 7–448.—Prominent fossa on lateral aspect of first cuneiform.

FIG 7–449.—**A** and **B,** central densities within the first cuneiform of a 3-year-old boy. **C** and **D,** appearance 1 year later.

FIG 7–450.—Bipartite first cuneiform on the patient's left foot (←). The right foot shows an os tibiale externum (⊬). The bipartite first cuneiform is more commonly divided into dorsal and plantar segments. (Ref: Kohler A, Zimmer EA: *Borderlands of the Normal and Early Pathologic in Skeletal Roentgenology,* ed 3. New York, Grune & Stratton, 1968, p 512.)

FIG 7–451.—Supernumerary bone arising from the left first cuneiform (←) on the right foot. It is represented by an osseous protuberance (⊬). (Ref: Rao B: Supernumerary toe arising from the medial cuneiform. *J Bone Joint Surg* 1979; 61A:308.)

FIG 7–452.—Supernumerary bones arising from the medial cuneiform.

FIG 7–453.—Unnamed ossicle above the first cuneiform.

FIG 7–454.—Simulated fracture produced by a well-demonstrated joint between the fourth metatarsal and the third cuneiform.

FIG 7–455.—Congenital fusion of the cuboid and the third cuneiform.

FIG 7–456.—**A,** simulated fracture of the cuboid. **B,** magnification view shows the simulated fracture is due to the dense cortex of the upper margin of the bone.

FIG 7–457.—Fossae in the posterior aspect of the cuboid, which should not be mistaken for erosions.

FIG 7–458.—Accessory bone of the lateral aspect of the distal end of the cuboid.

FIG 7–459.—The groove for the peroneus longus tendon.

FIG 7–460.—Overlapping shadows of cuboid and cuneiforms producing unusual shadow bilaterally.

FIG 7–461.—The os vesalianum, which lies in the peroneus longus tendon (see Fig 7–356). (Ref: Smith CD, et al: The os vesalianum: An unusual cause of lateral foot pain. *Orthopedics* 1984; 7:86.)

FIG 7–462.—Accessory ossification center at the distal end of the first metatarsal.

FIG 7–463.—Developmental notch in the distal end of the first metatarsal in a young child.

FIG 7–464.—Accessory ossification center of the distal end of the first metatarsal (→) in an 8-year-old boy with an epiphyseal spur (↠) (see Fig 6–239).

FIG 7–465.—Accessory ossification centers at the bases of the second, third, and fourth metatarsals. These are of no clinical significance.

FIG 7–466.—Accessory ossification centers at the bases of the second to fifth metatarsals with partial fusion in a 4-year-old boy.

FIG 7–467.—Accessory ossification centers at the bases of metatarsals 2 through 5 (←) and an accessory center at the distal end of the first metatarsal (↞) in a 12-year-old boy.

FIG 7–468.—Normal irregularities of the bases of the metatarsals in a 3-year-old boy.

FIG 7–469.—Duplication of the ossification center of the head of the third metatarsal, not a fracture.

FIG 7–470.—Duplication of the ossification center of the base of the first metatarsal.

FIG 7–471.—Oblique fissures in the metaphysis of the distal end of the first metatarsal, not to be mistaken for fractures.

FIG 7–472.—The normal apophysis of the tuberosity of the base of the fifth metatarsal, which resembles a fracture. Most fractures of this area are horizontal rather than vertical.

FIG 7–473.—Multicentric ossification centers of the tuberosities of the fifth metatarsals in a 12-year-old girl, simulating fractures.

FIG 7–474.—The lateral position of the apophysis of the base of the fifth metatarsal in the oblique projection should not be misconstrued as an avulsion injury.

FIG 7–476.—The fusing apophysis at the base of the fifth metatarsal may simulate a fracture in the frontal projection.

FIG 7–477.—Closing apophysis that might be mistaken for fracture at the base of the fifth metatarsal in an 11-year-old boy.

FIG 7–478.—Asymmetric closure of the apophysis of the base of the fifth metatarsals in an 11-year-old boy. *Top,* left foot. *Bottom,* right foot.

FIG 7–479.—Four examples of failure of union of the apophysis of the base of the fifth metatarsal in adults.

FIG 7–480.—Apophysis at the tip rather than at the side of the base of the fifth metatarsal in a 14-year-old boy. (Ref: Dameron JB: Fractures and anatomical variation of the proximal portion of the fifth metatarsal. *J Bone Joint Surg* 1975; 57A:788.)

FIG 7–481.—Bilateral closing apophyses of the type shown in Figure 7–480 in a 12-year-old boy that could be mistaken for a fracture. *Left and center*, left foot. *Right*, right foot.

FIG 7–482.—Unfused apophysis at the base of the fifth metatarsal in a 19-year-old man. Note that the apophysis is located at the end of the metatarsal rather than in its usual lateral position as in Figures 7–472 and 7–474. This is an unusual, but not rare, variation in the position of the apophysis.

FIG 7–483.—Asymmetric closure of the apophyses at the bases of the fifth metatarsals in a 20-year-old man.

FIG 7–484.—Very large apophyses at the bases of the fifth metatarsals in an 11-year-old boy.

FIG 7–485.—Closing apophysis at the base of the fifth metatarsal (←). Note how the trabeculations of the bone appear to line up in continuity with the apophyseal plate and simulate a fracture of the base (↔).

FIG 7–486.—Note the horizontal trabeculations in the base of the fifth metatarsal. It is these lines that create the illusion of horizontal fracture as shown in Figure 7–485.

FIG 7–487.—Duplication anomaly of the fifth metatarsal with nonunion of the basal apophysis *(arrow)*.

FIG 7–488.—Notch at the base of the fifth metatarsal that might be mistaken for evidence of fracture.

FIG 7–489.—Os vesalianum fused to base of fifth metatarsal (see Figs 7–357 and 7–461).

FIG 7–490.—Metatarsus adductus is physiologic in many infants and will correct spontaneously with weight-bearing. **A,** 4 months of age. **B,** 16 months of age. (Ref: Berg EE: A reappraisal of metatarsus adductus and skewfoot. *J Bone Joint Surg* 1986; 68A:1185.)

FIG 7–491.—Normal clefts seen at the bases of the metatarsals.

FIG 7–492.—Accessory ossicle at the base of the third metatarsal.

FIG 7–493.—Normal irregularity of the epiphyseal line at the base of the first metatarsal in an adolescent boy, which should not be mistaken for evidence of fracture.

FIG 7–494.—Three examples of normal irregularities of the bases of the second, third, and fourth metatarsals evident in oblique projection.

FIG 7–495.—Simulated torus fracture produced by the tuberosity of the base of the second metatarsal in a 13-year-old girl.

FIG 7–496.—Exaggeration of normal fossa in the head of the first metatarsal.

FIG 7–498.— Two examples of increase in size and cortical thickness of the shaft of the second metatarsal, seen in patients with short first metatarsals. This is apparently a compensatory weight-bearing mechanism.

FIG 7–497.—Developmental spur at the base of the third metatarsal.

FIG 7–499.—Two examples of the nutrient channel for the fourth metatarsal.

FIG 7–500.—Simulated fracture of the base of the fourth metatarsal, resulting from overlapping of the cuboid.

FIG 7–501.—Developmental cleft at the base of the fourth metatarsal in a young child.

FIG 7–502.—The os intermetatarseum. This accessory bone presents on the dorsal aspect of the foot and is variable in size and shape. It may be separate or attached to the base of the first or second metatarsal (see Fig 7–358). (Ref: Kohler A, Zimmer EA: *Borderlands of the Normal and Early Pathologic in Skeletal Roentgenology,* ed 3. New York, Grune & Stratton, 1968, p 523.)

FIG 7–503.—Os intermetatarseum arising from the base of the first metatarsal, unlike the example in Figure 7–502 that arose from the base of the second metatarsal.

FIG 7–504.—Bilateral os intermetatarseum.

FIG 7–505.—Variation in configuration of the os intermetatarseum.

FIG 7–506.—Fossa in the base of the second metatarsal secondary to the presence of a small os intermetatarseum.

FIG 7–507.— Simulated fracture of the first metatarsal, produced by the os intermetatarseum.

FIG 7–508.—Os intermetatarseum (→) and developmental fusion between the fourth and fifth metatarsal (→→).

FIG 7–509.—Unusual os intermetatarseum.

FIG 7–510.—The flat configuration of the head of the second metatarsal and resultant widening of the joint space should not be misconstrued as evidence of aseptic necrosis (Freiberg's disease). (Ref: Jenson EL, de Carvalho A: A normal variant simulating Freiberg's disease. *Acta Radiol* 1987; 28:85.)

FIG 7–511.— Accessory ossification centers in the distal ends of the first metatarsals in an 8-year-old boy.

FIG 7–512.—Bilateral symmetrical accessory ossification centers at the distal ends of the first metatarsals in an 11-year-old boy (←). Note clefts in the distal ends of the proximal phalanges as well (⇇).

FIG 7–513.—Partial closure of the physes of the fourth and fifth metatarsals in a 14-year-old girl.

FIG 7–515.—The dorsofibular process of the head of the first metatarsal, a normal variant. (Ref: Fischer E: Der dorsofibulare Fortsatz am Kopf des 1. Metatarsale, eine ossare Variante. *Radiologe* 1988; 28:45. Used by permission.)

FIG 7–514.—Closed accessory ossification center of distal end of the first metatarsal (←) with a dorsofibular process (see Fig 7–515).

FIG 7–516.—*Left,* deep cleft in the head of the fifth metatarsal in a 23-year-old woman in oblique projection. *(arrow). Right,* frontal projection shows unusual configuration of the head of the metatarsal.

FIG 7–517.—Exaggeration of the normal curvature of the fifth metatarsal.

FIG 7–518.—Developmentally short fifth metatarsal.

FIG 7–519.—Axial projection of the shafts of the proximal phalanges, simulating a cyst in the head of the fifth metatarsal.

FIG 7–520.—Anomalous articulation between the third and fourth metatarsals.

FIG 7–521.—Supernumerary metatarsal between the fourth and fifth metatarsals.

FIG 7–522.—Developing sesamoids in a 12-year-old boy, seen in lateral projection.

FIG 7–523.—Three examples of sesamoids at the distal interphalangeal joint of the first toe.

FIG 7–524.—Sesamoids at the second and fifth metatarsal heads.

FIG 7–525.—Bony ossicles, resembling sesamoids, on the dorsal aspect of both interphalangeal joints of the great toes in a 36-year-old woman.

FIG 7–526.—Sesamoid at the fifth metatarsophalangeal joint.

FIG 7–527.—Bipartite sesamoid of the first toe with unequal size of the members.

FIG 7–528.—Symmetric oval bipartite sesamoids of the first toe.

FIG 7–529.—Tripartite sesamoid of the first toe.

The Lower Extremity—The Sesamoid Bones **691**

FIG 7–530.—Multipartite sesamoid bone, simulating comminuted fracture.

FIG 7–531.—Multiple sesamoids of the metatarsal heads.

FIG 7–532 (left).—The sesamoid bones of the foot. (After Kohler A, Zimmer EA: *Borderlands of the Normal and Early Pathologic in Skeletal Roentgenology*, ed 3. New York, Grune & Stratton, 1968.)

FIG 7–533.—Fissure-like lucency in the sesamoids of the first toes, simulating fracture.

FIG 7–534.—Frontal and lateral projections of a bipartite sesamoid bone of the first toe with equal size of the members. (Ref: Feldman F, et al: The case of the wandering sesamoid and other sesamoid afflictions. *Radiology* 1970; 96:275.)

FIG 7–535.—Large sesamoid bone in the tibialis posterior tendon.

FIG 7–536.—Isolated sesamoid at the head of the third metatarsal.

FIG 7–537.—Divided epiphysis at the base of the proximal phalanx of the first toe, not a fracture. **A,** 3-year-old boy. **B,** 11-year-old boy. **C,** 13-year-old boy. (Ref: Lyritis C: Developmental disorders of the proximal epiphysis of the hallux. *Skeletal Radiol* 1983; 10:250.)

FIG 7–538.—Sixteen-year-old boy with cleft in the ossification center at the base of the proximal phalanx of the first toe in the plane opposite to that of Figure 7–537.

FIG 7–539.—**A** and **B,** bilateral cleft epiphyses of the proximal phalanx of the first toe. **C** and **D,** the appearance in the oblique projection could be mistaken for comminuted fracture.

FIG 7–540.—A, single ossification centers at the base of the first toe in an 11-year-old boy. B, 1 year later—the epiphysis has developed a cleft. This is a normal phenomenon that may be seen in any epiphysis (see Figs 6–129, 6–130, 7–123, and 7–283). (Ref: Harrison RB, Keats TE: The cleft epiphysis. *Skeletal Radiol* 1980; 5:23.)

FIG 7–541.—Development of cleft epiphysis. A, 3 years of age. B, 13 years of age.

FIG 7–542.—Bilateral persistence of the type of cleft epiphysis illustrated in Figure 7–541 into adult life.

FIG 7–543.—Fossa in the base of the proximal phalanx of the first toe possibly related to residuals of cleft epiphysis (see Fig 7–542).

FIG 7–544.—Cleft epiphysis of the base of the proximal phalanx of the second toe.

FIG 7–545.—Unusually deep fossae, bilaterally, at the bases of the proximal phalanges of the first toes.

FIG 7–546.—Fossa at the lateral aspect of the base of the proximal phalanx of the first toe with small ossicle within *(arrow)*. Note similarity to Figure 7–538.

FIG 7–547.—Normally dense epiphysis at the base of the proximal phalanx of the first toe in a 12-year-old boy. This should not be mistaken for evidence of osteochondrosis.

FIG 7–548.—Cone epiphyses are very common in the proximal phalanges of children and are not necessarily associated with abnormality.

FIG 7–549.—A, simulated fracture of the epiphysis of the first toe by oblique projection. **B,** no fracture seen in the frontal plane.

FIG 7–550.—*Left,* simulated fractures of the bases of the proximal phalanges in the oblique projection in an 11-year-old girl *(arrows). Right,* frontal projection shows no fractures. Note deep fossa in the head of the second metatarsal *(arrow).*

FIG 7–551.—Incomplete developmental fissures through the proximal phalanx of the first toe. **A,** 10-year-old boy. **B,** 12-year-old boy.

FIG 7–552.—Incomplete developmental fissure in the middle phalanx of the second toe in an 8-year-old boy.

FIG 7–553.—Fissures in the first, second, and third toes of a 10-year-old boy.

FIG 7–554.—Two examples of marked irregularity in development of the phalanges in 12-year-old girls. This is a normal and transient phenomenon.

FIG 7–555.—Developmental irregularity of the middle phalanx of the fourth toe in an 11-year-old girl, interpreted as a fracture.

FIG 7–556.—A, failure of fusion of a portion of the epiphysis at the base of the distal phalanx of the first toe, originally interpreted as a fracture despite absence of pertinent history or physical findings. **B,** 3-year follow-up shows no change.

FIG 7–557.—Three examples of ring-like defects seen near the joints of the toes. These represent small areas of fat necrosis, but are apparently of no importance clinically. (Ref: Keats TE, et al: Idiopathic punctate necrosis of the phalanges of the feet. *Skeletal Radiol* 1989; 18:25.)

FIG 7–558.—Two examples of spur-like enlargements of the distal phalanx of the great toe. They are of no clinical significance. *Right*, note the calcifications between the spurs that are located in the lateral supporting ligament. (Ref: Winter WG: Lateral supporting ligament of the distal phalanx. *Foot Ankle* 1989; 9:310.)

FIG 7–559.—Normal irregularities seen along the shafts of the proximal phalanges, not to be confused with periostitis.

FIG 7–560.—Two examples of fifth toes with only two phalanges. This is a common anatomic variant and not the product of disease. (Ref: Ellis R, et al: The two-phalanged fifth toe. *JAMA* 1968; 206:2526.)

FIG 7–561.— Two-phalanged third, fourth, and fifth toes, an anatomic variation.

FIG 7–562.—Pointed distal phalanges in a healthy 6-year-old girl.

FIG 7–563.—Pointed distal phalanges in a healthy 11-year-old boy. Absence of the distal tufts may be normal, unassociated with disease.

FIG 7–564.—Three examples of phalangeal sclerosis, a finding of no clinical significance. *Top left,* proximal phalanx. *Top right* and *bottom,* distal phalanges. (Ref: Carter BC, et al: Skeletal manifestations of idiopathic bone sclerosis. *Australas Radiol* 1988; 32:242.)

FIG 7–565.— Subungual calcification in the normal nail bed of the toes. This phenomenon is seen in adults in middle age and late life and is of no clinical significance. (From Fischer E: Subunguale Verkalkungen im normalen Nagelbett der Zehen. *Radiologe* 1984; 24:31–34. Used by permission.)

PART II

The Soft Tissues

Chapter 8

The Soft Tissues of the Neck

FIG 8–1.—Shadows of the lips seen in the frontal projection of the mandible.

FIG 8–2.—The pseudotumor of the nasal passage produced by superimposition of the coronoid process of the mandible on the inferior turbinate.

FIG 8–3.—Normal configuration of the soft tissues of the mouth and oropharynx in a 1-year-old infant during swallowing, showing tongue (→), soft palate (⇢), and adenoids (⇻).

FIG 8–4.—The shadow of the uvula seen in the basal view of the skull.

FIG 8–5.—The base of the tongue seen in the basal view of the skull.

FIG 8–6.—Large, but normal, adenoids in a young adult. The lucency within is due to superimposition of the nasopharyngeal air shadow.

FIG 8–7.—Air between the hard palate and the tongue.

FIG 8–8.—Calcification in the adenoids.

FIG 8–9.—The shadow of the ear lobe, simulating a mass in the nasopharynx.

FIG 8–10.—Hair braids simulating calcific thyroid mass.

FIG 8–11.—The ear lobe, simulating mass lesions, seen in preliminary films for submaxillary sialography.

FIG 8–12.—**A,** simulated soft tissue mass produced by the soft palate during phonation. **B,** same patient at rest. No mass present.

FIG 8–13.—A, pseudomass of the pharynx produced by the base of the tongue, filmed during the act of swallowing. **B,** normal configuration of soft tissues at rest in another patient for contrast with **A.**

FIG 8–14.—Prominent soft palate and uvula.

FIG 8–15.—The pharyngeal tonsil in a 3-year-old boy.

FIG 8–16.—Two examples of large pharyngeal tonsils, which may simulate a tumor of the pharynx.

FIG 8–17.—Calcification in the tonsilar crypts. (Ref: Aspestrand F, Kolben-stredt A: Calcifications of the palatine tonsillary region: CT demonstration. *Radiology* 1987; 165:479.)

FIG 8–18.—Normal alterations of the retropharyngeal soft tissues with respiration in infancy. **A,** quiet breathing. **B,** inspiration. **C,** expiration. The expiratory film resembles the changes of retropharyngeal abscess and is a potential source of misinterpretation.

FIG 8–19.—Two examples of normal prominence of the retropharyngeal soft tissues in expiration, misdiagnosed initially as retropharyngeal abscesses.

FIG 8–20.—Retropharyngeal soft tissue changes with respiration in a 1-year-old. *Left,* expiration. *Right,* inspiration.

FIG 8–21.—Thickening of the retropharyngeal tissues may also be seen in adults to a lesser degree. *Left,* inspiration. *Right,* expiration.

FIG 8–23.—Prominent prevertebral fat stripe, not to be mistaken for gas in the soft tissues. (Ref: Whalen JP, Woodruff CL: The cervical prevertebral fat stripe: A new aid in evaluating the cervical prevertebral soft tissue space. *AJR* 1970; 109:445.)

FIG 8–22.—Localized anterior bulging of soft tissues and impression on the posterior aspect of the trachea in an adult in expiration.

FIG 8–24.—Shadow of the glottis was originally misinterpreted as a fracture of the vertebral body.

FIG 8–25.—The styloid processes, which should not be mistaken for foreign bodies.

FIG 8–26.—Stylohyoid ligament calcification in an 11-year-old girl.

FIG 8–27.—Calcified stylohyoid ligaments in lateral (**A**) and oblique (**B**) projections.

FIG 8–28.—Extensively calcified stylohyoid ligaments in frontal (A) and lateral (B) projections (←). Note the articulation at the junction of the ligament and the styloid process (⫣). (Ref: Genez BM, et al: Case report 584: Ossified stylohyoid complex with pseudarthroses. *Skeletal Radiol* 1989; 18:623.)

FIG 8–29.—Calcified stylohyoid ligaments with multiple segments.

FIG 8–31.—Unilateral calcified stylohyoid ligament in an 11-year-old girl, mistaken for a foreign body.

FIG 8–30.—Partial calcification of the stylohyoid ligaments, simulating a foreign body.

FIG 8–33.—The hyoid bone in an 18-year-old woman. The synchondrosis between the body and greater cornua should not be mistaken for a fracture (→). Note also the lesser cornua (↠).

FIG 8–32.—Stylohyoid ligament calcification mistaken for impacted chicken bone.

FIG 8–34.—Simulated fracture of the hyoid in a 12-year-old girl.

FIG 8–35.—The arytenoid "bump."

FIG 8–36.—Variations in the arytenoid with phonation. **A,** quiet breathing. **B,** phonation.

FIG 8–37.—Calcification in the thyrohyoid ligament.

FIG 8–38.—Calcification in the arytenoid cartilage. (Ref: Jurik AG: Ossification and calcification of the laryngeal skeleton. *Acta Radiol Diagn* 1984; 25:17.)

FIG 8–39.—Calcification of the thyroid cartilages, simulating carotid artery calcification.

FIG 8–40.—Calcification of the entire thyroid cartilage.

FIG 8–41.—Calcification of the superior cornua of the thyroid cartilage, which might be mistaken for a foreign body.

FIG 8–42.—Calcification in the arytenoid cartilages (→). Note also a submaxillary gland calculus (↠). The *lowest arrow* indicates calcification in the posterior lamina of the cricoid cartilage (⫲).

FIG 8–43.—Calcification of the cricoid cartilages.

FIG 8–44.—**A,** calcification of the posterior cricoid lamina when seen in isolation may be easily confused with a foreign body. **B,** in a patient with more extensive calcification of the larynx, the relationship to the density seen in **A** is more easily identified.

FIG 8–45.—*Left,* unusually long tubular calcification arising from the cricoid cartilage and descending anteriorly and inferiorly. *Right,* CT shows the same structure. The nature of this variant is unknown. (From Nidecker A, et al: The cricoid cartilage: Observations on some roentgen variants. *ORL J Otorhinolaryngol Relat Spec* 1982; 44:170. Used by permission.)

FIG 8–46.—Physiologic calcification of the soft tissues of the neck. The *upper arrow* indicates calcification in the thyrohyoid ligament (cartilago triticea). The *middle arrow* shows calcification in the arytenoid cartilage. The *lower arrow* indicates calcification in the tracheal cartilage.

FIG 8–47.—Calcified arytenoid (←) and calcification of tracheal cartilages (⇎) in a 37-year-old woman.

FIG 8–48.—Physiologic calcifications in the frontal projection: thyroid cartilage (→), cartilago triticea (→), hyoid bone (�ît), and carotid artery calcification (⇸).

FIG 8–49.—Very dense calcification of the thyroid cartilages.

FIG 8–50.—Variations in appearance of the normal closed glottis in frontal projection.

FIG 8–51.—The suprasternal fossa in a newborn infant may simulate the distended proximal pouch of an esophageal atresia. (Ref: Hernandez R, et al: The suprasternal fossa on chest radiographs in newborns. *AJR* 1978; 130:745.)

FIG 8–52.—The suprasternal fossa in older children (**A**) or thin adults (**B** and **C**) may be quite deep and may cast a radiolucency that may be mistaken for an air-filled esophageal diverticulum. (Ref: Ominsky S, Berinson HS: The suprasternal fossa. *Radiology* 1976; 122:311.)

FIG 8–53.—Simulated gas in soft tissues produced by the suprasternal fossa.

FIG 8–54.—Simulated interstitial air in the neck posteriorly simulated by hair braids.

Chapter 9

The Soft Tissues of the Thorax

FIG 9–1.—Hair braids simulating gas in the soft tissues of the neck.

FIG 9–2.—Plastic hair braids producing unusual appearance of the soft tissues of the neck and shoulders.

FIG 9–3.—Simulated parenchymal lesions due to hair braids (←). Note similar shadow laterally on right (↤).

FIG 9–4.—Simulated pneumothorax in a 3½-year-old child due to a skin fold.

FIG 9–5.—The dense juvenile breast may cast shadows simulating parenchymal density (→). Note also shadows cast by hair braids (↦).

FIG 9–6.—Intersecting shadows of the breast (←) and pectoral folds (↤).

FIG 9–7.—Skin folds producing curvilinear densities in the lower thorax and upper abdomen in a 3-week-old infant.

FIG 9–8.—Folds of lax skin in the elderly may also simulate a pneumothorax.

FIG 9–9.—Four examples of skin folds simulating pneumothoraces. The patient illustrated in **D** was intubated. Note the fading margin of the skin fold in contrast to the sharp pleural line seen with a true pneumothorax. (Ref: Fisher JK: Skin fold versus pneumothorax. *AJR* 1978; 130:791.)

FIG 9–10.—Axillary folds simulating pneumothorax.

FIG 9–11.—Shadow of the descending aorta simulating localized pneumothorax.

FIG 9–12.—Redundant soft tissues of the axilla, producing rounded densities in the mediastinum.

FIG 9–13.—Nonsignificant asymmetry of the companion shadows of the clavicles, resulting from faulty positioning. No shadow is seen on the left side.

FIG 9–14.—Calcification in the costoclavicular fascia, not to be mistaken for parenchymal lesions. A, plain film. B, laminagraphy.

FIG 9–15.—Calcified costal cartilage may simulate a parenchymal lesion. **A,** plain film. **B,** laminagraphy.

FIG 9–16.—Exuberant calcified costal cartilage at the end of the first rib may produce mass effect behind the sternum in the anterior mediastinum. **A,** plain film. **B,** laminagraphy in the lateral projection shows that the mass consists of the calcified cartilage (→). Note position of trachea for orientation (⇥).

FIG 9–17.—Ring shadow of calcified costal cartilage of first rib simulating a cavity in lung.

FIG 9–18.—Simulated nodule produced by underdevelopment of the anterior end of the first rib with isolated development of the costal cartilage. *Left,* plain film. *Right,* tomogram.

FIG 9–19.—The floor of the supraclavicular fossa may be very well defined and simulate an air-fluid level in the lung. (Ref: Christensen EE, Dietz GW: The supraclavicular fossa. *Radiology* 1976; 118:37.)

FIG 9–20.—The confluence of the shadows of the sterno-cleidomastoid muscle, the first rib, and the clavicle may simulate a bulla or cavity in the apex of the lung.

FIG 9–21.—Two examples of the shadows of the subcostal muscles that produce an appearance simulating pleural thickening or small pneumothorax.

FIG 9–22.—Companion shadows of the ribs.

FIG 9–23.—Triangular companion shadow of the first rib.

FIG 9–24.—Congenital absence of the left pectoralis major muscle, producing increased radiolucency of the left hemithorax.

FIG 9–25.—Shadow of the pectoralis major muscle, simulating a lung lesion (←). Note also the pseudopneumothorax on the right, produced by a skin fold (↤).

FIG 9–26.—Extrapleural fat in a very obese man, simulating pleural thickening. The absence of blunting of the costophrenic angles in this entity is a useful differential clue. (Refs: Vix VA: Extrapleural costal fat. *Radiology* 1974; 112:563; and Sargent EN, et al: Subpleural fat pads in patients exposed to asbestos: Distinction from non-calcified pleural plaques. *Radiology* 1984; 152:273.)

FIG 9–27.—Additional example of extrapleural fat deposits in a very obese patient, simulating pleural thickening. The shadow of the extrapleural fat does not reach the costophrenic angles. Occasionally these extrapleural fat deposits may be slightly asymmetric. (Ref: Friedman AC, et al: Asbestos-related pleural disease and asbestosis: A comparison of CT and chest radiography. *AJR* 1988; 150:269.)

FIG 9–28.—Extrapleural fat seen in an off-lateral projection. Note that it loses its prominence at the bases.

FIG 9–29.—The serratus anterior muscle produces a shadow that may be confused with pleural thickening or extrapleural fat. In frontal views, it produces a "bowling pin" configuration. (Ref: Gilmartin D: The serratus anterior muscle on chest radiographs. *Radiology* 1979; 131:629.)

FIG 9–30.—Two additional cases showing the varying appearance of the serratus anterior muscle shadows.

FIG 9–31.—A demonstration of the muscle slips of the serratus anterior muscle that constitute the "bowling pin" sign.

FIG 9–32.—**A,** simulated parenchymal density produced by soft tissues over the scapula due to improper positioning of the arms. **B,** shadow not seen with proper positioning. (Ref: Lams PM, Jolles H: The scapula companion shadow. *Radiology* 1981; 138:19.)

FIG 9–33.—In an improperly positioned chest film, the spine of the scapula may overlap the lungs and produce a shadow that may be mistaken for a pneumothorax. (Ref: Harbin WP, Cimmino CV: The radiographic innominate lines of the scapular spine. *Va Med* 1974; 101:1050.)

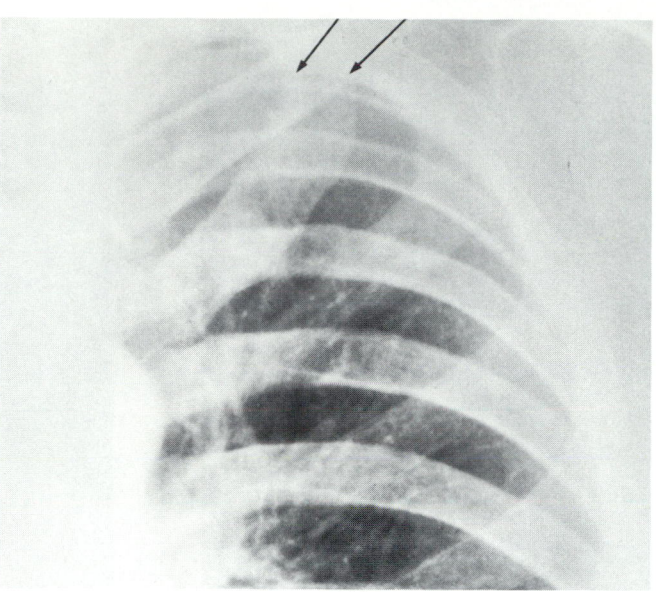

FIG 9–34.—End-on visualization of the anterior end of the first rib, simulating a pneumothorax.

FIG 9–35.—Lucency of medullary cavity of the second rib, simulating a pneumothorax.

FIG 9–36.—Two examples of the mammary anterior mediastinal pseudotumor. The lateral aspects of the dense, small breasts in young women may project into the anterior mediastinum in the lateral projection and simulate a mediastinal mass. (Ref: Keats TE: Mammary anterior mediastinal pseudotumor. *J Can Assoc Radiol* 1976; 27:262.)

FIG 9–38.—The compressed breast in the prone position may simulate a pneumothorax.

FIG 9–37.—The axillary tail of the breast may simulate an anterior mediastinal mass.

FIG 9–39.—Three examples of the sternal insertion of the pectoralis major muscle that might be mistaken for carcinoma on mammography. *Top,* triangular area of increased density is seen in medial aspect of breast on craniocaudal view (⊬), continuous with underlying pectoral muscle (←). *Center,* rounded area of increased density is seen in medial aspect of breast on craniocaudal view (←). *Bottom,* craniocaudal view of left breast in a female weightlifter reveals continuity between pectoral muscle (⊬) and density (←). (From Britton CA, et al: Carcinoma mimicked by sternal insertion of the pectoral muscle. *AJR* 1989; 153:955. Used by permission.)

FIG 9–40.—Prosthetic mammary implants. Note the similarity in this patient's lateral projection to the pseudotumor in Figure 9–36.

FIG 9–41.—Simulated air in soft tissues produced by rotation.

FIG 9–42.—Air under the breast, producing a striking radiolucency beneath the heart shadow in the lateral projection.

FIG 9–43.—The manubrium of a 2½-year-old boy, simulating a soft tissue mass.

FIG 9–44.—Simulated pneumothorax in a neonate produced by a skin fold. **A,** simulated pneumothorax. **B,** normal appearance 5 hours later.

FIG 9–45.—Subcostal muscle, simulating pleural thickening *(left)* or pneumothorax *(right)*.

FIG 9–46.—Blunted costophrenic angles in children and young adults are often seen as an apparently normal, incidental, and inconsistent finding that many times cannot be reproduced on the same day. It is frequently misinterpreted as evidence of pathologic pleural effusion or pleuritis. It may be due to redundancy of the pleura or may represent the pleural fluid normally present in the pleural space in healthy children and possibly in young adults. (Ref: Ecklof O, Torngren A: Pleural fluid in healthy children. *Acta Radiol [Diagn]* 1971; 11:346.)

FIG 9–47.—A, simulated intrapulmonary effusion as evidenced by increased distance between the stomach air bubble and the dome of the diaphragm. B, the apparent separation is due to the marked posterior position of the fundus of the stomach with projection of the diaphragm above.

FIG 9–48.—Triangular area of relative obliteration of the diaphragm, said to be due to extension of areolar tissue into the base of the inferior pulmonary ligament. (Ref: Proto AV, Speckman JM: The left lateral radiograph of the chest. *Med Radiogr Photogr* 1979; 55:69.)

FIG 9–49.—Four examples of the aortic pulmonary stripe, a reflection of the mediastinal pleura from the aorta to the pulmonary artery. This should not be confused with displacement of the mediastinal pleura due to adenopathy. (From Keats TE: The aortic-pulmonary mediastinal stripe. *AJR* 1972; 116:107. Used by permission.)

FIG 9–50.—Six examples of azygos lobes to demonstrate the variation in configuration of the pleural line (←) and the position and size of the azygos vein (⫢).

FIG 9-51.—Additional examples of azygos lobes to demonstrate the variation in configuration of the pleural line (←) and the position and size of the azygos vein (↔).

FIG 9-52.—The azygos lobe and arch and its continuity with the azygos vein *(arrows).*

FIG 9-53.—The lingular fissure. This fissure separates the lingula from the remainder of the left upper lobe (←). It duplicates the minor fissure on the right (╫). (Ref: Boyden EA: Cleft left upper lobes and the split anterior bronchus. *Surgery* 1949; 26:167.)

FIG 9–54.—Two examples of an accessory fissure of the left upper lobe, the left azygos lobe. (Ref: Takasugi JE, Goodwin JD: Left azygos lobe. *Radiology* 1989; 171:133.)

FIG 9–55.—The superior accessory fissure of the left lower lobe. This fissure separates the superior and basal segments of the left lower lobe. A similar fissure occurs in the right lower lobe. (Ref: Felson B: The lobes and interlobar pleura. Fundamental roentgen considerations. *Am J Med Sci* 1955; 230:572.)

FIG 9–56.—Superior accessory fissure by plain film *(left)* and with pneumothorax *(right)*.

FIG 9–57.—Cephalic curvature of the minor interlobar fissure may be seen as a normal variation.

FIG 9–58.—Accessory fissure for the superior segment of the right lower lobe. Note the presence of two pleural lines in the frontal projection. (Ref: Godwin JD, Tarver RD: Accessory fissures of the lung. *AJR* 1985; 144:39.)

FIG 9–60.—The superimposed scapular spines may simulate interlobar pleural surfaces.

FIG 9–59.—The minor fissure may normally be seen posteriorly and may be mistaken for the accessory fissure seen in Figure 9–58.

FIG 9–61.—The inferior accessory fissure. When complete, it isolates the medial basal segment of the lower lobe. (Ref: Felson B: The lobes and interlobar pleura. Fundamental roentgen considerations. *Am J Med Sci* 1955; 230:572.)

FIG 9–62.—Sagittal orientation of the minor fissure. Note how it may simulate pneumopericardium. (Ref: Gross BH, et al: Sagittal orientation of the anterior minor fissure: Radiography and CT. *Radiology* 1988; 166:717.)

FIG 9–63.—The vertical fissure line. This line represents the caudal end of the major interlobar fissure. It may be seen in films of healthy children when it is ectopic and lies forward so part of it is in axial projection. It should not be mistaken for a pneumothorax. (Ref: Davis LA: The vertical fissure line. *AJR* 1960; 84:451.)

FIG 9–64.—The vertical fissure line. **A,** unilateral. **B,** bilateral. (Ref: Webber MM, O'Loughlin BJ: Variations of the pleural vertical fissure line. *Radiology* 1964; 82:461.)

FIG 9–66.—Pleural reflection over the inferior vena cava. A, apparent paraspinous mass (←) produced by pleural reflection over the inferior vena cava (⊣⊢). B, detailed view with greater penetration shows no paraspinous mass.

FIG 9–65.—The vertical fissure line with extension over the apex of the right lower lobe.

FIG 9–67.—The esophageal pleural stripe that represents the right esophageal wall and its adjacent pleural covering. A, plain film. B, esophagram. (Ref: Cimmino CV: The esophageal-pleural stripe on chest teleroentgenograms. *Radiology* 1956; 67:754.)

FIG 9–68.—The posterior mediastinal stripe, the interface of the right and left lungs, seen in frontal projection. (Ref: Cimmino CV, Snead LO Jr: The posterior mediastinal line on chest roentgenograms. *Radiology* 1965; 84:516.)

FIG 9–69.—The posterior mediastinal line seen in its entirety.

FIG 9–70.—The anterior mediastinal stripe, representing the interface between the right and left lungs, seen in frontal projection (←). The posterior mediastinal stripe is also evident (⊬). (Ref: Cimmino CV: The anterior mediastinal line on chest roentgenograms. *Radiology* 1964; 82:459.)

FIG 9–71.—The anterior mediastinal stripe and its lateral extensions.

FIG 9–72.—Two examples of simulated pneumothorax in neonates, produced by skin folds.

FIG 9–73.—Bulging of the interspaces in a normal child. Although intercostal bulging of the lung is said to be an early sign of obstructive emphysema, it may also be seen in normal, thin children who inspire fully. (Ref: Kattan KR, et al: Intercostal bulging of the lung without emphysema. *AJR* 1971; 112:542.)

FIG 9–74.—The scapulae seen in lordotic projection may simulate pulmonary pathology (←), particularly the shadow of the spine of the scapula (⇔).

FIG 9–75.—Films made of infants in isolettes may show radiolucencies due to the opening in the isolette covers. These may simulate abnormalities such as air cysts, as in **A,** or pneumopericardium, as in **B.**

FIG 9–76.—Two examples of hair braids simulating parenchymal abnormality.

FIG 9–77.—Filming infant chests in even minor degrees of expiration may result in misinterpretation due to the marked opacity of the parenchyma, as illustrated in this normal infant. **A,** expiration. **B,** inspiration.

FIG 9–78.—Filming in expiration may simulate basal pneumonitis in the adult. **A,** inspiration. **B,** expiration.

FIG 9–79.—Simulated air trapping in the right middle lobe. This misleading appearance is not infrequent and results from the pattern of division of the major vascular trunks. There is no evidence of air trapping in the lateral projection. (Refs: Milne ENC, Bass H: The right midlung window. *J Can Assoc Radiol* 1969; 20:3; and Goodman LR, et al: The right midlung window. *Radiology* 1982; 143:135.)

FIG 9–80.—The effects of respiration on the trachea in infancy. The trachea (←) widens on inspiration (**A**) and narrows on expiration (**B**). The *hatched arrows* (⇤) in **B** indicate swallowed air in the esophagus. Note also the normal anterior buckling of the airway in the neck on expiration. (Ref: Wittenberg MH, et al: Tracheal dynamics in infants with respiratory distress, stridor, and collapsing trachea. *Radiology* 1967; 88:613.)

FIG 9–81.—Tracheal narrowing on expiration in a 3-week-old infant, illustrating how marked this physiologic event may normally be.

FIG 9–82.—*Left*, portable chest films that are made with lordotic projection will produce an illusory consolidation of the left lower lobe with loss of the medial portion of the left hemidiaphragm. *Right*, film made with proper projection does not show the pseudoconsolidation. (Ref: Zylak CJ, et al: Illusory consolidation of the left lower lobe: A pitfall in portable radiology. *Radiology* 1988; 167:653.)

The Soft Tissues of the Thorax—The Lungs   757

FIG 9–83.—Normal anterior tracheal indentation in a 2-year-old child. This is a common finding just below the thoracic inlet, is believed to be vascular in origin, and is usually of no clinical significance. (Ref: Swischuk LE: Anterior tracheal indentation in infancy and early childhood: Normal or abnormal? *AJR* 1971; 112:12.) This entity may be seen in 30% of normal children under the age of 2 years. (Ref: Stripe JL, et al: Tracheal compression by the innominate artery in infancy and childhood. *Radiology* 1981; 139:73.)

FIG 9–84.—A shallow impression on the right side of the trachea at the thoracic inlet is seen in many normal children (**A**) and adults (**B**).

FIG 9–85.—Lateral buckling of the trachea at the thoracic inlet occurs normally in infants and children up to 5 years of age. The displacement is to the side opposite the aortic arch and is best seen in expiration. (Ref: Chang LWM, et al: Normal lateral deviation of the trachea in infants and children. *AJR* 1970; 109:247.)

FIG 9–86.—Deviation of the trachea to the left in the presence of a right aortic arch.

FIG 9–87.—A, tracheal buckling on expiration in an adult. B, inspiration does not show buckling.

FIG 9–88.—Normal anterior bowing of the trachea in the adult, associated with ectasia of the aorta.

FIG 9–89.—Calcification of the tracheal and bronchial cartilagenous rings in a 47-year-old healthy woman. This is unusual except in old age unless the patient has hypercalcemia or hyperphosphatemia.

FIG 9–90.—Expiratory film with superimposition of the right hemidiaphragm on the heart, producing an image simulating atelectasis of the right middle lobe.

FIG 9–91.—Two examples of large transverse processes that simulate nodular pulmonary lesions.

FIG 9–92.—Large hypertrophic spur simulating a parenchymal lesion in both frontal and lateral projections.

FIG 9–93.—Hypertrophic spurs simulating lung nodules.

FIG 9–94.—Hypertrophic spur simulating lung nodule. *Left*, lateral projection. *Right*, CT.

FIG 9–95.—*Left,* large transverse process simulating lung nodule. *Right*, film made with slight rotation does not reproduce the pseudonodule.

FIG 9–96.—Two examples of hypertrophy of interarticulating facets producing pseudonodules.

FIG 9–97.—Soft tissues of the arm seen in lateral projection, simulating atelectasis of the upper lobe.

FIG 9–98.—Prominent nipple shadow in male, simulating a nodular pulmonary lesion.

FIG 9–99.—Nipple shadows may cause confusing images in the lateral projection in poorly positioned patients.

FIG 9–100.—Skin lesions may produce nodular shadows that simulate parenchymal nodules, in this case a large nevus.

FIG 9–101.—Two examples of simulated cavitary lesions produced by superimposition of vascular shadows. This phenomenon is common in the perihilar areas.

FIG 9–102.—Pseudolesion of lung produced by superimposition of normal upper lobe vascular structures on the arch of the aorta (see Fig 9–125). (Ref: Stark P, et al: Pseudolesion of the chest: A conglomerate shadow on the lateral radiograph. *Chest* 1985; 87:541.) (See also Fig 9–125.)

FIG 9–103.—The rhomboid fossa of the clavicle simulating a cavitary lesion of the right upper lobe.

FIG 9–104.—The shadows of the subclavian arteries may simulate a pleural or parenchymal density.

FIG 9–105.—Bilateral apical opacities probably produced by the subclavian arteries. (Ref: Proto AV, Chaliff MI: Apical opacity: A normal finding on posteroanterior chest radiography. *Radiology* 1986; 161:429.)

The Soft Tissues of the Thorax—The Lungs

FIG 9–106.—Films made in expiratory phases of respiration show greater prominence of the pulmonary arteries (→) and the confluence of the pulmonary veins (⇢). Note also the vascular prominence in the posterior base in **A** (⇤). The shadow of these vessels is often misinterpreted as evidence of pneumonitis. The problem does not present itself in films made with good inspiration, as in **B.**

FIG 9–107.—The pulmonary veins in lateral projection may assume a somewhat nodular configuration.

FIG 9–108.—The confluence of the pulmonary veins at the left atrium may present as a nodular density, which should not be confused with a mass lesion. **A,** plain frontal film. **B,** oblique projection. **C,** frontal laminagram. **D,** lateral laminagram.

FIG 9–109.—The confluence of the pulmonary veins.

FIG 9–110.—The scimitar vein, an anomalous vessel that drains into the inferior vena cava below the diaphragm. This vein may be an isolated finding, as in this case, or associated with hypoplasia of the right lung. (Ref: Roehm JO Jr, et al: Radiographic features of the scimitar syndrome. *Radiology* 1966; 86:856.)

FIG 9–111.—"Physiologic" calcification of the tracheobronchial cartilages in a 56-year-old woman.

FIG 9–112.—Mucus plugs in the trachea may simulate significant lesions, such as neoplasms. **A,** laminagram of the trachea, showing filling defect. **B,** laminagram after coughing up mucus plug. (Ref: Karasick D, et al: Mucoid pseudotumors of the tracheobronchial tree in two cases. *AJR* 1979; 132:459.)

FIG 9–113.—Arterial shadow superimposed on the bronchus, simulating a broncholith.

FIG 9–114.—Vertebral hypertrophic spurs may simulate pulmonary lesions.

FIG 9–115.—**A,** the azygos lobe may simulate an infiltrate in a standard frontal film. **B,** same area seen in lordotic projection, showing the usual appearance of the azygos lobe.

FIG 9–116.—Normal variability in size of the bronchi at bronchography, dependent on the degree of filling with iodized oil.

FIG 9–117.—Variations in bronchial branching; the accessory cardiac bronchus. (Ref: Mangulea VG, Stinghe RV: The accessory cardiac bronchus. *Dis Chest* 1968; 54:433.)

FIG 9–118.—Variations in branching of the right upper lobe bronchus. **A,** normal. **B,** agenesis of the right upper lobe bronchus. The upper lobe is supplied by the intermediate bronchus. (Ref: Lafret EG, et al: Anomalies of upper lobe bronchial distribution. *J Thorac Cardiovasc Surg* 1962; 43:595.)

FIG 9–119.—Two examples of duplication of the right upper lobe bronchus. The upper branch supplies the apical segment. (Refs: Harris JH: The clinical significance of the tracheal bronchus. *AJR* 1958; 79:228; and Ritsema GH: Ectopic right bronchus: Indication for bronchography. *AJR* 1983; 140:671.)

FIG 9–120.—A, the tracheal bronchus seen on plain film. B, CT showing tracheal bronchus. C, CT cut below B, at level of the tracheal bifurcation.

FIG 9–121.—Arm fold superimposed on anterior mediastinum, producing a mass effect. (Ref: Vaezy A, Delaney DJ: Chest wall mass mimicking pulmonary tumor. *South Med J* 1979; 72:499.)

FIG 9–122.—The scapula and arm fold producing a simulated lucent mass.

FIG 9–123.—A, superimposition of a rib shadow on the aortic arch simulates an air-fluid level. B, the top of the arch of the aorta may simulate an air-fluid level in the esophagus.

FIG 9–124.—The spine of the scapula simulating a cavitary lesion with air-fluid level.

FIG 9–125.—Superimposition of the shadows of the aorta and scapula produces a triangular shadow of increased density (see Fig 9–102).

FIG 9–126.—The angle of the scapula, simulating a lung nodule.

FIG 9–127.—Examples of the retrosternal line produced by the interface between the two lungs and the mediastinal fat. (Ref: Whalen JP, et al: The retrosternal line. A new sign of an anterior mediastinal mass. *AJR* 1973; 117:861.)

FIG 9–128.—*Left*, prominent retrosternal line. *Right*, CT shows the mechanism of production of the line. The right lung extends to the anterior chest wall. The left lung is excluded by the heart and mediastinal fat *(arrow)*. The difference in anterior extension of the two lungs creates the retrosternal line.

FIG 9–129.—**A,** unusually prominent retrosternal line produced by rotation at the time of filming. **B,** true lateral shows more usual appearance.

FIG 9–130.—Very prominent retrosternal line.

FIG 9–131.—Superimposition of the ribs and the retrosternal line, producing a factitious mass.

FIG 9–132.—In some individuals with well-defined retrosternal lines, an additional line (the right parasternal stripe) may be seen through the right side of the heart. This line indicates the medial edge of the right lung. (Ref: Keats TE: The right parasternal stripe: A new mediastinal shadow and a contribution to the nature of the retrosternal line. *AJR* 1974; 120:898.)

FIG 9–133.—Three examples of clinically unimportant triangular radiolucencies in the anterior mediastinum in adults. The mechanism of production of these shadows is not proved, but they are probably the result of the same anatomy that produces the retrosternal line, illustrated in Figure 9–127.

FIG 9–134.—Five examples of triangular anterior mediastinal radiolucencies seen in young children with large thymuses. They may represent the same entity illustrated in Figure 9–133 or are possibly related to the presence of the thymus. (Ref: Quattromani FL, et al: Fascial relationship of the thymus. *AJR* 1981; 137:1209.)

FIG 9–135.—Manubrial ossification centers in an infant, which may be confused with mediastinal masses.

FIG 9–136.—A, simulated pneumomediastinum produced by sternal retraction. **B,** follow-up examination shows normal appearance.

FIG 9–137.—The manubrium, simulating a mediastinal mass (←) produced by slight scoliosis. The azygos arch is seen below (⇍).

FIG 9–138.—The anterior extrapleural line represents a deviation of the pleura produced by the innominate artery and vein and the costal cartilages of the first ribs. It should not be mistaken for a lesion of the sternum or a mediastinal mass. (Ref: Whalen JP, et al: Anterior extrapleural line: Superior extension. *Radiology* 1975; 115:525.)

FIG 9–139.—The anterior extrapleural line in a child, misinterpreted as a mass lesion. **A,** conventional film. **B,** xerogram.

—Two examples of mediastinal fat, producing widening of the mediastinum. This may be seen in obesity, in Cushing's disease, and in patients receiving steroids. (Ref: Price JE Jr, Rigler LG: Widening of the mediastinum resulting from fat accumulation. *Radiology* 1970; 96:497.) Seen in lateral projection, such fat may simulate the thymus. (Ref: Steckel RJ: Mediastinal pseudotumors associated with exogenous obesity. *Radiology* 1976; 119:74.)

FIG 9–141.—CT, showing extensive mediastinal lipomatosis.

FIG 9–142.—Alterations in configuration of the mediastinum over a period of 25 years due to mediastinal deposition of fat. An azygos lobe is present.

FIG 9–143.—Progressive mediastinal lipomatosis over a 10-year period secondary to steroids. Note displacement of the aortic pulmonary stripe in (**B**) (←).

FIG 9–144.—Mediastinal lipomatosis with marked displacement of the aortic pulmonary stripe.

FIG 9–145.—Mediastinal fat simulating a dilated ascending aorta *(arrows)*.

FIG 9–146.—Fat seen in anterior mediastinum with increase over 2-year period with progressive obesity.

FIG 9–147.—Mediastinal lipomatosis. Note also extension of the fat over the apex of the lungs and into the extrapleural spaces *(arrows)*.

FIG 9–148.—*Left*, confusing appearance produced by mediastinal lipomatosis (←) and an azygos lobe (↔). *Right*, CT shows the course of the azygos vein.

FIG 9–149.—A, widening of the right side of the mediastinum due to distention of the superior vena cava after forceful Valsalva maneuver. **B,** same patient in suspended respiration without Valsalva maneuver.

FIG 9–150.—An azygos lobe simulating a distended air-filled esophagus. **A,** plain film. **B,** laminagraphy.

FIG 9–151.—Widening of the superior vena cava due to anomalous venous drainage of the left upper lobe. The anomalous vertical vein is evident. (Ref: Adler SC, Silverman JF: Anomalous venous drainage of the left upper lobe. *Radiology* 1973; 108:563.)

FIG 9–152.—The spurious posterior mediastinal mass, seen in infants as the result of superimposition of the scapulae and the axillary soft tissues, combined with the anterior curve of the trachea and the lower lobe continuation of the left main bronchus. (Refs: Alazraki NP, Friedman PJ: Posterior mediastinal "pseudo-mass" of the newborn. *AJR* 1972; 116: 571; and Balsand D, et al: The scapula as a cause of spurious posterior mediastinal mass on lateral chest films of infants. *J Pediatr Surg* 1974; 9:501.)

FIG 9–153.—The pseudomass of the mediastinum in infants, illustrated in Figure 9–152, will be accentuated by filming in the expiratory phase of respiration. **A,** expiration. **B,** full inspiration. No mass effect seen.

FIG 9–154.—The normal paravertebral stripe. Note that it is not normally seen in the upper thoracic region, being lost at T4–5. This is best seen in the patient on the right.

FIG 9–155.—The normal left paravertebral soft tissues. *Arrow* indicates the paravertebral stripe; *crossed arrow* indicates the descending aorta. (Ref: Lien HH, Kolbenstvedt A: The thoracic paraspinal shadow: Normal appearances. *Clin Radiol* 1982; 33:31.)

FIG 9–156.—The left paramediastinal stripe (→), representing the reflection of the pleura against the spine, may be deviated laterally by ectasia of the thoracic aorta (↠) and is, therefore, not necessarily an indication of vertebral or mediastinal abnormality. (Ref: Genereux GP: The posterior pleural reflections. *AJR* 1983; 141:141.)

FIG 9–157.—The paravertebral stripe may be seen on the right, particularly in young individuals (**A** and **B**), or bilaterally (**C**) and should not be confused with a paraspinous mass. A similar shadow on the right may also be due to a wide inferior vena cava. (Ref: Eklof O, et al: Malignant versus benign paravertebral widening in children. *Pediatr Radiol* 1981; 11:193.)

FIG 9–158.—Right and left paravertebral stripes in a 49-year-old woman.

FIG 9–159.—Displacement of the right paravertebral stripe by hypertrophic lipping of the spine.

FIG 9–160.—A very narrow chest will result in striking visualization of both paravertebral stripes.

FIG 9-161.—Paraspinous fat deposition will displace the paravertebral stripes. **A,** plain film. **B,** CT. (Refs: Streiter ML, et al: Steroid-induced thoracic lipomatosis: Paraspinal involvement. *AJR* 1982; 139:679, and Glickstein MC, et al: Paraspinal lipomatosis. *Radiology* 1987; 163:79.)

FIG 9-162.—*Left,* striking paraspinal lipomatosis that is bilaterally symmetric. *Right,* CT.

FIG 9-163.—Marked obesity resulting in displacement of the paravertebral stripe, due to fat deposition. **A,** 300-lb 14-year-old boy. **B,** 250-lb 46-year-old man.

FIG 9–164.—The paraspinous fat deposits may not be evenly distributed or symmetric, as illustrated in this case. *Left,* plain film. *Right,* CT.

FIG 9–165.—Origin of the psoas muscles from the lower thoracic spine, producing paraspinous soft tissue shadows.

FIG 9–166.—Thoracic origin of very large psoas muscles, producing paravertebral soft tissue bulges. **A** and **B**, frontal projections. **C** and **D**, oblique projections.

FIG 9–167.—Four examples of discrete, unexplained left paravertebral soft tissue bulges that have not been explained by CT or aortography. They appear to be unimportant and may be related to the hemiazygous system. (Ref: Castellino RA, et al: Dilated azygous and hemiazygous veins presenting as paravertebral intrathoracic masses. *N Engl J Med* 1968; 278:1087.)

FIG 9–168.—**A,** simulated pneumomediastinum is evidenced by radiolucency adjacent to the aorta, produced by lucent lung in the interval between the aorta and adjacent pulmonary vessels. **B,** with slight rotation to the left, the nature of this factitial lesion is evident.

FIG 9–169.—A, simulated pneumomediastinum evidenced by a lucent halo around the heart due to the Mach effect. **B,** no evidence of pneumomediastinum in lateral projection. (Ref: Friedman AC, et al: Mach bands and pneumomediastinum. *J Can Assoc Radiol* 1981; 32:232.)

FIG 9–170.—Simulated pneumomediastinum in an infant, produced by slight rotation of the chest at the time of filming, projecting lucent lung in front of the cardiac shadow.

FIG 9–171.—Air in the esophagus producing a lucency beneath the aortic arch (←). This is seen when the esophagus is displaced to the left by adhesions to a tortuous aorta. Barium may be retained in this pocket as well. Note position of pleural esophageal reflection (⊬). (Ref: Cimmino CV: A roentgenologic study in mediastinal anatomy affected by air in the midesophagus. *AJR* 1965; 94:333.)

FIG 9–172.— Three examples of patients with transient reflux of gas in the esophagus that should not be confused with mediastinal gas. (Ref: Proto A, Lane KJ: Air in the esophagus: A frequent radiographic finding. *AJR* 1977; 129:433.)

FIG 9–173.—**A** and **C**, examples of air trapped in the midesophagus (→) as in Figure 7–172. Note in **A** that the shift of the esophagus to the left has permitted a portion of the right lung to cross the left side, producing an additional area of radiolucency (→). **B**, the barium esophagram of the patient shown in **A**. Note that the knuckle in the aorta corresponds to the air shadow in the plain film. (Ref: Proto AV: Air in the esophagus: A frequent radiologic finding. *AJR* 1977; 129:433.)

FIG 9–174.—The azygos arch may be seen in the lateral projection as a nodular density, immediately behind the trachea. **A,** child. **B,** adult.

FIG 9–175.—The shadows of the normal azygos vein. **A,** the arch of the azygos vein. **B,** the posterior portion of the azygos arch, the "azygos knob." **C,** the posterior portion of the azygos arch by laminagraphy. (Ref: Heitzman ER, et al: The azygous vein and its pleural reflections. *Radiology* 1971; 101:259.)

FIG 9–176.—The azygos knob may be seen without tomography.

FIG 9–177.—On tomography, the azygos knob may simulate an intratracheal mass. (Ref: Austin JHM, Thorson MK: Normal azygous arch: Retrotracheal visualization on frontal chest tomograms. *AJR* 1981; 137:1205.)

FIG 9–178.—The azygopulmonary recess (→). *Hatched arrow* (↤) indicates the posterior portion of the azygos arch.

FIG 9–179.—The azygos arch seen in lateral projection by tomography.

FIG 9–180.—In congenital absence of the inferior vena cava with azygous continuation, the arch of the azygous is large and may be mistaken for a mediastinal mass. (Refs: Heller RM, et al: A useful sign in the recognition of azygous continuation of the inferior vena cava. *Radiology* 1971; 101:519; and Pallin J, et al: Azygous continuation of the inferior vena cava masquerading as neoplasm. *South Med J* 1989; 82:259.)

FIG 9–181.—Proportional difference between the size of the heart and thorax in a newborn and an adult. The heart in infancy occupies a proportionately larger area of the thorax than it does in the adult, and adult criteria for heart size cannot be applied to infants and children. (From Keats TE: Pediatric radiology: Some potentially misleading variations from the adult. *Va Med* 1966; 93:630. Used by permission.)

FIG 9–182.—Normal variability in heart size with changes in cardiac cycle in a child. **A,** systole. **B,** diastole.

FIG 9–183.—Normal variability in heart size with changes in cardiac cycle in an adult. **A,** systole. **B,** diastole.

FIG 9–184.—*Left,* heart movements during filming may produce a confusing double contour of the left heart border, representing systole (←) and diastole (↤). *Right,* the same effect may be seen during laminagraphy in another patient.

FIG 9–185.—Decrease in heart size resulting from Valsalva effect. *Left,* baseline. *Right,* after Valsalva maneuver.

FIG 9–186.—The shadows of the bronchus and pulmonary vessel, adjacent to the right heart border, simulate pneumopericardium.

FIG 9–187.—A large thymus, simulating cardiomegaly. Note the normal heart size in the lateral projection.

FIG 9–188.—Very small hearts are not necessarily of significance and are often seen in young, asthenic women. (Ref: Swischuk LE: Microcardia: An uncommon diagnostic problem. *AJR* 1968; 103:115.)

FIG 9–189.—Pseudomyocardial aneurysm of the posterior wall of the left ventricle. **A,** a discrete bulge is seen on the posterior wall of the left ventricle that is not seen in an exposure made later in the same session **(B).** This bulge is seen fluoroscopically and shows apparent paradoxic movement. It represents a transient phase of contraction of the left ventricle late in systole and is a normal phenomenon. (From Keats TE, Martt JM: False paradoxic movement of the posterior wall of the left ventricle simulating myocardial aneurysm. *Radiology* 1962; 78:381. Used by permission.)

FIG 9–190.—Additional example of the pseudoaneurysm of the posterior wall of the left ventricle.

FIG 9–191.—Four examples of the visualization of the right border of the left atrium in normal children. This may be seen also in adults and should not be taken as evidence of left atrial enlargement in itself, unless correlative evidence is present in the other projections. (Ref: Rosario-Medina W, et al: Normal left atrium: Appearance in children on frontal chest radiographs. *Radiology* 1986; 161:345.)

FIG 9–192.—Elevation of the cardiac apex in a normal 2-year-old child produced by very deep inspiration. This configuration should not be confused with the alteration due to ventricular hypertrophy.

FIG 9–193.—The subepicardial fat line seen as a lucent crescent beyond the heart shadow (←). The pericardium (⊹) is sandwiched between this fat line and the fat in the mediastinum. (Ref: Lane EJ Jr, Carsky EW: Epicardial fat: Lateral plain film analysis in normals and in pericardial effusion. *Radiology* 1968; 91:1.)

FIG 9–194.—Subepicardial fat, which could be mistaken for pneumopericardium, seen in frontal and lateral projections in a 7-year-old boy. (Ref: Kremens V: Demonstration of pericardial shadow on routine chest roentgenogram: A new roentgen finding. *Radiology* 1955; 64:72.)

FIG 9–195.—Visualization of the pericardium at the right heart border in a 4-year-old boy on two different occasions. Its visualization is due to the presence of subepicardial fat. The pericardial shadow should not be misinterpreted as calcification in the pericardium. (Ref: Keats TE: Four normal anatomic variations of importance to radiologists. *AJR* 1957; 78:89.)

FIG 9–196.—Normal cardiac changes in pregnancy. **A,** in addition to cardiac enlargement, there is a rather selective dilatation of the right atrium in some normal women during pregnancy. In addition, the arch of the azygos vein enlarges (←). **B,** regression of these changes shortly after parturition. (Refs: Keats TE, Martt JM: Selective dilatation of the right atrium in pregnancy. *AJR* 1964; 91:307; and Keats TE, et al: Mensuration of the azygous vein and its application to the study of cardiopulmonary disease. *Radiology* 1968; 90:990.)

FIG 9–197.—The straight back syndrome, producing flattening of the heart and prominence of the pulmonary artery. Individuals with congenital absence of the normal dorsal kyphosis and narrow sagittal diameter of the chest present striking alterations in cardiac contour compounded by the coexistence of physical findings that may mimic organic heart disease. (Ref: de Leon A, et al: The straight back syndrome. *Circulation* 1965; 17:197.)

FIG 9–198.—The straight back syndrome, showing distortion of the aortic arch and descending aorta.

FIG 9–199.—Normal epipericardial fat pads. These fat collections may be confused with cysts and neoplasms. They vary in size with the weight of the patient. (Ref: Holt JF: Epipericardial fat shadows in differential diagnosis. *Radiology* 1947; 48:472.)

FIG 9–200.—Unusual configuration of epipericardial fat pad.

FIG 9–201.—Small, discrete, round epipericardial fat pad in the right cardiophrenic angle.

FIG 9–202.—Additional examples of epipericardial fat pads. (Ref: Nahon JR: Roentgen characteristics of the epipericardial fat pad with a case report. *Radiology* 1955; 65:745.)

FIG 9–203.—Increasing size of epipericardial fat pad over a 6-year period with progressive obesity.

FIG 9–204.—Extension of the epipericardial fat pad into the major interlobar fissure. (Ref: Gale ME, Greif WL: Intrafissural fat: CT correlation with chest radiography. *Radiology* 1986; 160:333.)

FIG 9–205.—Two examples of triangular shadows at the lung base produced by extension of the epipericardial fat pad into the left major fissure anteriorly (←) and the shadow of the inferior vena cava posteriorly (⟵).

FIG 9–206.—Extension of an epipericardial fat pad into the minor interlobar fissure.

FIG 9–207.—Irregular epipericardial fat pad misinterpreted as a neoplasm and removed by thoracotomy (→).
A, plain film, lateral view. Note extension into the major interlobar fissure. (↤). **B,** tomogram.

FIG 9–208.—*Left,* baseline film. *Right,* 10 years later right middle lobe atelectasis was misdiagnosed due to superimposition of epipericardial fat pad with extension into the major interlobar fissure *(arrow).*

FIG 9–209.—Unusual configuration of epipericardial fat pad, showing increasing size over a 1-year period with increasing obesity.

FIG 9–210.—Lucency under the heart due to pressure of epipericardial fat.

FIG 9–211.—Normal, but prominent, azygos arch in a young adult. This structure can be distinguished from an enlarged azygos node by noting its change in size between the supine and upright positions. (Ref: Keats TE, et al: Mensuration of the arch of the azygous vein and its application to the study of cardiovascular disease. *Radiology* 1968; 90:990.)

FIG 9–212.—Marked dilatation of the arch of the azygos vein in congenital interruption of the inferior vena cava. Note absence of a shadow of the inferior vena cava in the lateral projection. This sign is not always useful in diagnosis, since it may not be seen in some normal individuals. (Ref: Heller R, et al: A useful sign in recognition of azygous continuation of the inferior vena cava. *Radiology* 1971; 101:519.)

FIG 9–213.—The shadow of the left subclavian artery in a 75-year-old man (←). The edge of the manubrium is seen on the opposite side (⊬).

FIG 9–214.—Marked calcification in the great vessels.

FIG 9–215.—Mass effect due to dilated brachiocephalic vessels (→) and arm shadow (⇸).

FIG 9–216.—A, broadened mediastinal outline on the left due to a very large left subclavian artery (→). An azygous lobe is present (⇇). B, CT shows the large artery.

FIG 9–217.—Three examples of the aortic nipple. This normal shadow is due to the highest intercostal vein and is seen in children and adults. (Ref: Ball JB Jr, Proto AV: The variable appearance of the left superior intercostal vein. *Radiology* 1982; 144:445.) The nipple should not exceed 4.5 mm in diameter. (Ref: Friedman AC, et al: The normal and abnormal left superior intercostal vein. *AJR* 1978; 131:599.)

FIG 9–218.—Three examples of the ductus bump in neonates. This density is seen in normal infants in the first day of life and usually disappears by the third day. It represents a reflection of neonatal adjustment to extrauterine life and is the shadow of the ductus functioning briefly before closure. (Ref: Berdon WE, et al: The ductus bump: A transient physiologic mass in chest roentgenograms in newborn infants. *AJR* 1965; 95:91.)

FIG 9–219.—The infundibulum of the ductus, the point of insertion of the ductus in early life. Its presence does not indicate patency of the ductus. (Ref: Keats TE, Steinbach HL: Patent ductus arteriosus: A critical evaluation of its roentgen signs. *Radiology* 1955; 64:528.) The infundibulum may produce a figure-of-3 configuration, as illustrated in this case, that should not be misinterpreted as evidence of coarctation of the aorta or aortic rupture. (Refs: Yousefzadeh DK, et al: The aortic isthmus. *Radiology* 1981; 140:710; and Morse SS, et al: Atypical ductus diverticulum mistaken for aortic rupture. *AJR* 1988; 150:753.)

FIG 9–220.—Calcification in the ligamentum arteriosum.

FIG 9–221.—Four examples of normal variation in size of the pulmonary artery in children and young adults. The pulmonary artery is extremely variable in size, and its prominence in the young is a common finding. It should not be a source of concern in itself. **A,** 5-year-old boy. **B,** 8-year-old boy. **C,** 9-year-old girl. **D,** 18-year-old boy.

FIG 9–222.—The right aortic arch (→) with retroesophageal course is not necessarily associated with congenital heart disease and may be mistaken for a mediastinal mass. It displaces the esophagus to the left and anteriorly (⇸).

FIG 9–223.—**A,** tortuous aorta presenting on the right heart border *(arrows)*. **B,** lateral projection shows tortuosity.

FIG 9–224.—**A,** widened mediastinum in this acutely injured patient is due to filming in expiration and was misinterpreted as evidence of aortic rupture. **B,** inspiratory film made within an hour of **A** shows normal appearance.

FIG 9–225.—Normal widening of the mediastinal silhouette in the supine position. This finding coupled with buckling of the aorta to the right in expiration (←) may lead to an erroneous diagnosis of traumatic rupture of the aorta (see Figure 9–87). **A,** upright. **B,** supine.

FIG 9–226.—Lateral displacement of the superior vena cava by an ectatic aortic arch. (Ref: Drasin E, et al: Nondilated superior vena cava presenting as a superior mediastinal mass. *J Can Assoc Radiol* 1972; 23:273.)

FIG 9–227.—Three examples of left superior vena cava.

FIG 9–228.—Idiopathic dilatation of the superior vena cava is a developmental variant of no significance. **A,** plain film. **B,** tomogram. **C,** angiocardiogram. (Ref: Polansky S, et al: Idiopathic dilatation of the superior vena cava in children. *Pediatr Radiol* 1974; 2:167.)

FIG 9–229.—Another example of idiopathic dilatation of the superior vena cava. Note similarity to preceding case.

FIG 9–230.—A prominent, but normal, shadow of the inferior vena cava.

FIG 9–231.—Idiopathic dilatation of the inferior vena cava, so-called varix of the inferior vena cava, a finding of no clinical significance in itself. (Ref: Oh KS, et al: Inferior vena cava varix. *Radiology* 1973; 109:161.)

FIG 9–232.—Three examples of confusing radiolucencies produced by the inferior vena cava. With maximum inspiration, it is possible to clear a portion of the diaphragmatic surface of the heart and expose the anterior wall of the inferior vena cava (→). This results in a triangular area of radiolucency (⇢), which may be confusing if its origin is not appreciated. (Ref: Tonkin IL, et al: Radiographic isolation of the inferior vena cava. *AJR* 1977; 129:657.)

FIG 9–233.—Shadow of the inferior vena cava, producing an appearance simulating atelectasis.

FIG 9–234.— Variations in the configuration of the thymus. **A,** at birth, an appearance simulating configuration of the thymus seen in pneumomediastinum. **B,** the same individual at 16 months. The thymus is still prominent, but more closely applied to the mediastinum.

FIG 9–235.— Three examples of unilateral presentation of the thymus to the right side.

FIG 9–236.—Two examples of the thymic wave sign. The undulating configuration of the edge of the thymus is due to impression of the anterior portion of the ribs. (Ref: Mulvey RB: The thymic "wave" sign. *Radiology* 1963; 81:834.)

FIG 9–237.—Two examples of large left lobes of the thymus producing an appearance suggesting dextrocardia.

FIG 9–238.—Two examples of very large thymuses simulating cardiomegaly.

FIG 9–239.—Unilateral presentation of the thymus to the right and extending almost to the diaphragm.

FIG 9–240.—Huge thymus at 9 months of age.

FIG 9–241.—Huge thymus simulating cardiomegaly in the frontal plane. Note the radiolucency on the right in contrast to the heart on the left.

FIG 9–242.—A, large thymus simulating cardiomegaly. B, the lateral projection fails to show corresponding cardiomegaly and indicates the large thymic outline anteriorly. C and D, dextro- and levo-angiocardiograms show normal cardiac size within the huge thymus.

FIG 9–243.—The left lobe of the thymus simulating enlargement of the left atrial appendage.

FIG 9–244.—Unilateral "sail" configuration of the right lobe of the thymus.

FIG 9–245.—Unusual configuration of the thymus. Note the large shadow of the thymus in the lateral projection.

FIG 9–246.—Unusually rounded configuration of the thymus.

FIG 9–247.—Two examples of the thymus producing an appearance resembling the "snowman heart" of total anomalous pulmonary venous return.

FIG 9–248.—Examples of the thymus presenting entirely to the right side.

FIG 9–249.—The thymus in a neonate, producing a relative radiolucency anteriorly in the lateral projection, which was originally mistaken for a hernia through Morgagni's foramen.

FIG 9–250.—Right lobe of the thymus simulating right upper lobe pneumonitis. The thymus may simulate upper lobe atelectasis as well. (Ref: Lanning P, Heikkinen E: Thymus simulating left upper lobe atelectasis. *Pediatr Radiol* 1980; 9:177.)

FIG 9–252.—Posterior mediastinal thymus, a rare variant. At surgery the thymus was connected to the anterior mediastinum by a thin pedicle. (Refs: Cohen MD, et al: The diagnostic dilemma of the posterior mediastinal thymus: CT manifestations. *Radiology* 1983; 146:691: Bar-Ziv J, et al: Posterior mediastinal accessory thymus. *Pediatr Radiol* 1984; 14:165; and Siegel MJ, et al: Normal and abnormal thymus in childhood: MR imaging. *Radiology* 1989; 172:367.)

FIG 9–253.—The thymus does not always regress in early childhood and may persist into early adolescence. Its presence in late childhood, therefore, should not be construed as evidence of abnormality. Note residual thymus in a 4-year-old boy. (Ref: Oh KS, et al: Normal mediastinal mass in late childhood. *Radiology* 1971; 101:625.)

FIG 9–254.—Late persistence of the thymus. **A,** age 1 year. **B,** age 9 years.

FIG 9–255.—Residual thymus in a 6-year-old girl.

FIG 9–256.—Residual thymus in a 6-year-old boy.

FIG 9–257.—A, residual thymus in an 8-year-old girl. **B,** 2-year follow-up.

FIG 9–258.—Residual thymus in a 9-year-old boy.

FIG 9–259.—Residual thymus in a 9-year-old boy, which can be traced across the mediastinum.

FIG 9–260.—Residual thymus in an 11-year-old boy. **A,** frontal projection. Frontal (**B**) and left anterior oblique (**C**) projections

FIG 9–261.—Residual thymus in a 13-year-old girl.

Chapter 10

The Diaphragm

Pages
829 to **834**

Figures
10–1 to **10–15**

FIG 10–1.—The sternal insertions of the diaphragm, which consist of a pair of short, narrow slips that arise from the back of the xiphoid and pass backward to be inserted into the central tendon of the diaphragm. (Ref: Kleinman PK, Raptopoulos V: The anterior diaphragmatic attachments. *Radiology* 1985; 155:289.)

FIG 10–2.—"Scalloping" of the diaphragm is caused by hypertrophy and contraction of individual muscle bundles in the diaphragm. This case shows multiple small convexities.

FIG 10–3.—"Scalloping" of the diaphragm with several large convexities.

FIG 10–4.—"Scalloping" of the diaphragm.

FIG 10–5.—Additional variations of "scalloped" diaphragms.

FIG 10–6.—High insertions of the medial attachments of the diaphragm, simulating mass lesions. **A,** inspiration. **B,** partial expiration, in which the attachments are not seen as clearly.

FIG 10–7.—Muscular slips of the diaphragm seen in maximal inspiration.

FIG 10–8.—Localized eventration of the diaphragm in a child. Without benefit of the lateral projection, this variation could be mistaken for a mass lesion.

FIG 10–9.—Localized eventration of the posterior aspect of the diaphragm.

FIG 10–10.—Intrathoracic migration of the right kidney through the right foramen of Bochdalek in a 70-year-old woman that was not present on an examination made 20 years previously. Diaphragmatic defects and pseudolesions such as fat or visceral herniations through diaphragmatic defects increase in number and severity in the seventh and eighth decades. (Ref: Laskey CI, et al: Aging of the diaphragm: A CT study. *Radiology* 1989; 171:385.)

FIG 10–11.—Intrathoracic migration of the kidney through the foramen of Bochdalek not seen on shallow inspiration *(left)*, but visualized with maximum inspiration *(right)*.

FIG 10–12.—Bilateral anterior diaphragmatic eventration in a newborn. This condition may be asymptomatic. Note upward displacement of the heart. (Ref: Avnet NE: Roentgenologic features of congenital bilateral anterior diaphragmatic eventration. *AJR* 1962; 88:743.)

FIG 10–13.—The increased distance between the stomach gas bubble and the diaphragm suggests a subpulmonic effusion. The lateral projection indicates that this appearance is due to the fact that the posterior portion of the left hemidiaphragm (→) is higher than the anterior portion (↠), which is adjacent to the gas bubble.

FIG 10–14.—Increased distance between the stomach gas bubble and the diaphragm in lateral projection due to the medial position of the gas bubble (←) in relation to the highest point of the dome of the diaphragm (↞).

FIG 10–15.—Increased distance between the stomach gas bubble and the diaphragm in lateral projection due to the impression of the heart on the gas bubble *(arrows).*

Chapter 11

The Soft Tissues of the Abdomen

FIG 11–1.—Skin folds in an infant, producing an unusual appearance of the hepatic shadow.

FIG 11–2.—Posterior skin folds in an elderly patient, lending a striking appearance to the abdomen.

FIG 11–3.—A, simulated lucency of the psoas muscles due to folding of the soft tissues of the back. B, this appearance is not seen in the subsequent film after alteration of the patient's position.

FIG 11–4.—Simulated mass in the right flank produced by muscle splinting on that side.

FIG 11–5.—Skin fold, simulating a lucent psoas shadow.

FIG 11–6.—Lucent stripes in the shadow of the psoas muscle due to fat between the msucle bundles.

FIG 11–7.—Two examples of simulated pneumoperitoneum due to Mach effect of the rib superimposed on the diaphragm.

FIG 11–8.—Simulated pneumoperitoneum due to subdiaphragmatic fat. (Ref: Rao KG, Woodlief RM: Excessive right subdiaphragmatic fat: A potential diagnostic pitfall. *Radiology* 1981; 138:15.)

FIG 11–9.—Fat may also be seen beneath the left hemidiaphragm, as illustrated in these two cases.

FIG 11–10.—**A,** fat between the fundus of the stomach and the diaphragm. **B,** the lateral projection shows fat anteriorly beneath the diaphragm.

FIG 11–11.—Simulated pneumoperitoneum due to fat between the fundus of the stomach and the diaphragm. *Top,* two air-fluid levels are seen in the upright frontal film. *Arrow* (←) indicates fat; *hatched arrow* (⟻) indicates stomach. *Bottom,* the lateral projection shows anterior position of the stomach with a large air-fluid level (↠) and fat interposed between the stomach and the diaphragm (→). Note how far anteriorly the normal stomach may extend.

FIG 11–12.—Simulated pneumoperitoneum due to fat between the junction of the stomach and the diaphragm.

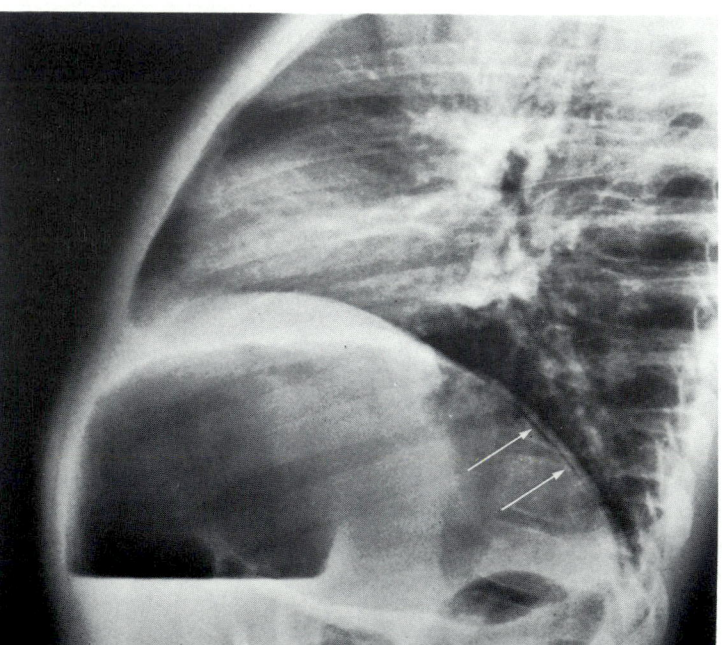

FIG 11–13.—Simulated pneumoperitoneum produced by lucent interval between the two diaphragmatic shadows and an air-filled stomach.

FIG 11–15.—Simulated air-fluid level beneath the right hemidiaphragm, resulting from through projection of the different heights of the base of the diaphragm (→) and its dome (↠).

FIG 11–14.—**A** and **B,** simulated pneumoperitoneum with an air-fluid level (→), which appeared to be distant from the stomach air bubble. **C** and **D,** the problem is clarified by inflating the stomach with more air, indicating that both gas collections are in the stomach. The apparent separation in **B** is the result of the two diaphragmatic contours (⫶).

FIG 11–16.—Air beneath the breasts, simulating pneumoperitoneum.

FIG 11–17.—Simulated pneumoperitoneum produced by fat around the lateral and superior aspect of the liver. The right side of the liver may also be visualized by ascites. (Ref: Proto AV, Lane EJ: Visualization of differences in soft-tissue densities. *Radiology* 1976; 121:19.)

FIG 11–18.—CT showing the fat around the liver that produces the radiolucency seen in Figure 11–17.

FIG 11–19.—Colonic interposition on the right, simulating pneumoperitoneum.

FIG 11–20.—Colonic interposition simulating pneumoperitoneum in the frontal film.

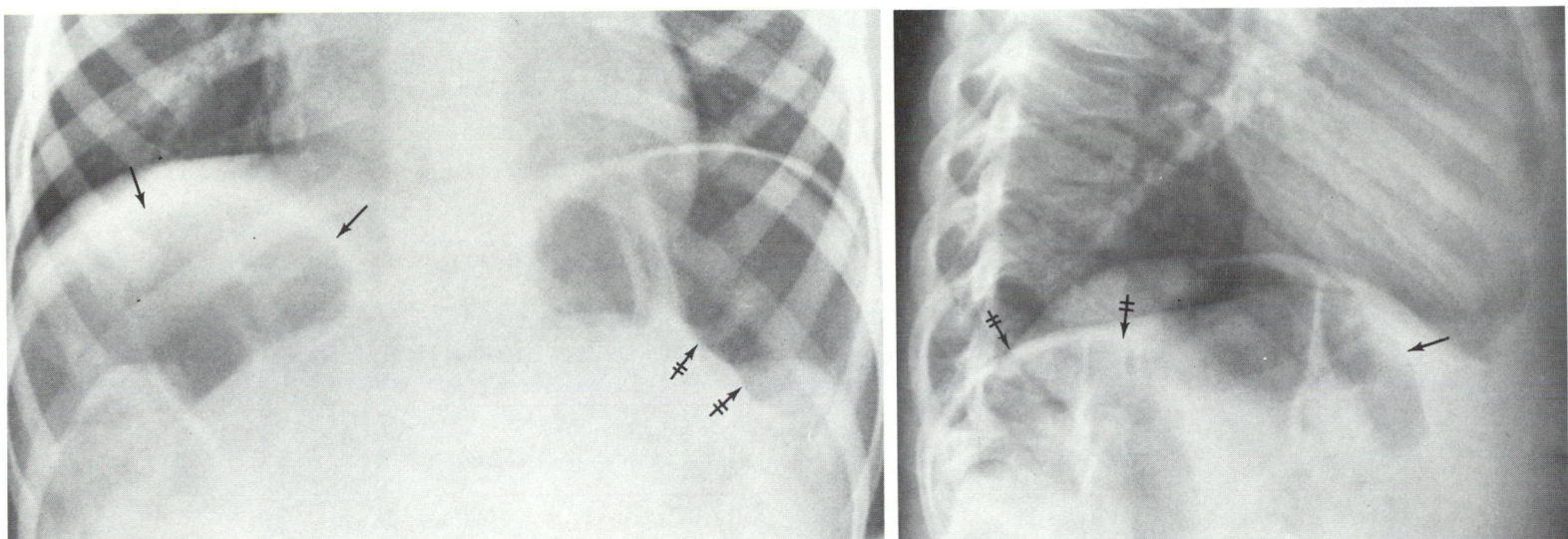

FIG 11–21.—Colonic interposition between the liver and the diaphragm (←) and between the spleen and the diaphragm (╫) in a 3-year-old child. This is a common finding in children and is not usually productive of symptoms. It should not be confused with pneumoperitoneum. (Ref: Behlke FM: Hepatodiaphragmatic interposition in children. *AJR* 1964; 91:669.)

FIG 11–22.—Colonic interposition between the liver and diaphragm in a 4-year-old boy (**A**) and its spontaneous reduction on the same day (**B**).

FIG 11–23.—Colonic interposition, simulating a subphrenic abscess. **A,** supine film. **B,** upright film.

FIG 11–24.—In the supine position, the fluid-filled fundus of the stomach simulates a mass lesion. *Left,* plain film; *right,* laminagraphy. This pseudotumor may opacify on angiography and thus further obscure its proper identification. (Ref: Bjorn-Hansen RW, O'Brien DS: Aortographic opacification of the gastric fundus simulating neoplasm. *AJR* 1967; 100:408.)

FIG 11-25.—A, the fluid-filled duodenal bulb may present as a right upper quadrant mass in the prone position. B, supine position shows mass less distinctly. C, barium examination shows the mass effect to be due to the duodenal bulb.

FIG 11-26.—A, in the prone position the fluid-filled gastric antrum may also simulate a right upper quadrant mass. B, antrum filled with barium in same position as A. (Ref: Balthazar E: Right upper quadrant pseudotumor, a fluid-filled viscus. *Radiology* 1974; 112:11.)

FIG 11–27.—The gas-filled gastric fundus displacing the shadow of the spleen *(arrows)* from the diaphragm, simulating a mass.

FIG 11–28.—The left lobe of the liver presenting into the stomach gas bubble, simulating a neoplasm (see Fig 11–71).

FIG 11–29.—The liver shadow encroaching on the stomach gas bubble in both projections.

FIG 11–30.—Fluid-filled splenic flexure of the colon, simulating a mass encroaching on the stomach.

FIG 11–31.—Posterior lung margins, simulating abdominal mass.

FIG 11–32.—Simulated properitoneal fat line produced by the contact of the patient's arm with the abdomen (←). A true properitoneal fat line is seen on the opposite side (↤).

The Soft Tissues of the Abdomen—The Abdomen in General **847**

FIG 11–33.—Fat around the ligamentum teres of the liver, producing a bilobed appearance of the liver or a simulated mass. (Ref: Haswell DM, et al: Plain film recognition of the ligamentum teres hepatis. *Radiology* 1975; 114:263.)

FIG 11–34.—Riedel's lobe of the liver, which may be mistaken for a right lower quadrant mass (see Fig 11–179).

FIG 11–35.—Riedel's lobe of the liver (→) and perinephric fat (↦) produce an appearance suggesting gas in the perirenal space.

FIG 11–36.—Two examples of the double wall sign. The ability to see both sides of the bowel wall is not reliable evidence of pneumoperitoneum. In these cases, it is due to two loops of distended intestine in contact with each other. (Ref: deLacy G, et al: Pneumoperitoneum, the misleading double wall sign. *Clin Radiol* 1977; 28:445.)

FIG 11–37.—Extensive mesenteric fat simulating pneumoperitoneum.

FIG 11–38.—Air in the appendix is a normal phenomenon and should not be considered as evidence of acute appendicitis. (Refs: Shimkin PM: Radiology of acute appendicitis. *AJR* 1978; 130:1001; and Shaffer HA, Harrison RB: Gas in the appendix. *Arch Surg* 1979; 114:587.)

FIG 11–39.—The shadow of the umbilicus seen in the oblique projection of the abdomen.

FIG 11–40.—Gastric contents, simulating the changes of bronchiectasis at the base of the left lung.

FIG 11–41.—Visualization of the diaphragmatic attachments.

FIG 11–42 (left).—Ring-shaped calcified costal cartilage, simulating gallstones.

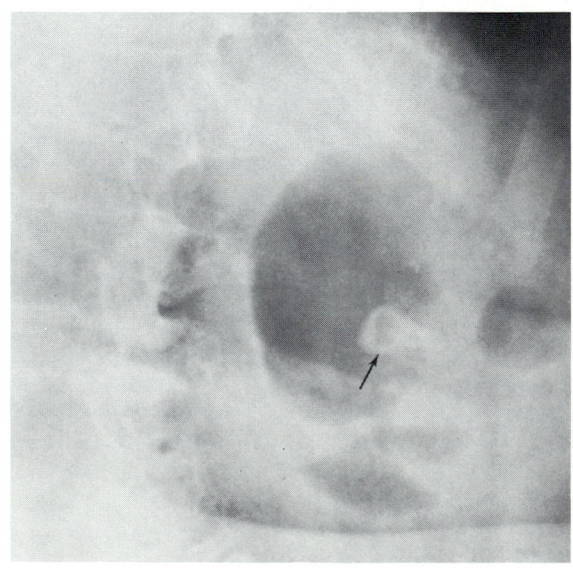

FIG 11–43 (right).—Calcified costal cartilage in the left upper quadrant, simulating a renal calculus.

FIG 11–44.—Calcification in a tortuous splenic artery.

FIG 11–45.—Ingested seeds in the transverse colon, simulating pancreatic calcification.

FIG 11–46.—Enteroliths in the cecum formed about ingested prune pits.

FIG 11–47.—The ossification center of the last coccygeal segment in a 10-year-old boy, which should not be mistaken for a calculus.

FIG 11–48.—Dystrophic calcification in obliterated umbilical arteries in a 2-year-old child, an unusual normal finding in infants. (From Currarino G, Weinberg A: Dystrophic calcification in obliterated umbilical artery. *Pediatr Radiol* 1985; 15:346. Used by permission.)

FIG 11–49.—The edge of the sacroiliac joint simulating calcification in the appendix. The appearance is less marked on the opposite side.

FIG 11–50.—The lingual tonsil, which consists of a fine fibrous network, containing lymphoid tissue scattered over the pharyngeal part of the tongue. (Ref: Gromet NL: Lymphoid hyperplasia in the base of the tongue. *Radiology* 1982; 144:825.)

FIG 11–52.—The impression of the cricopharyngeus muscle.

FIG 11–53.—Four examples of the variable appearance of the postcricoid impression, which is due to the prolapse of lax mucosal folds over the ventral submucosal venous plexus *(arrows)*. It is not seen after the barium bolus is passed. (Ref: Pitman RG, Frazer GM: The postcricoid impression on the esophagus. *Clin Radiol* 1965; 16:34.)

FIG 11–54.—Marked shift of the esophagus to the left at the thoracic inlet due to narrowness of the bony inlet. This variation is often confused with displacement by a mass lesion. (Ref: Kendall BE, et al: A physiologic variation in the barium-filled gullet. *Br J Radiol* 1962; 35:769.)

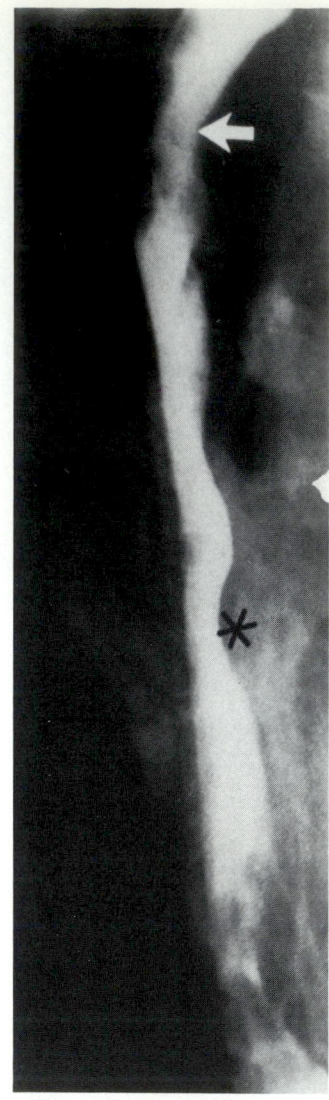

FIG 11–55.—Pulmonary venous indentation on the esophagus, caused by pressure of the inferior pulmonary vein, a normal variant. The *asterisk* indicates the venous impression; the *arrow* marks the aortic arch. (From Yeh H-C, Wolf BS: A pulmonary venous identation on the esophagus—a normal variant. *Radiology* 1975; 116:299. Used by permission.)

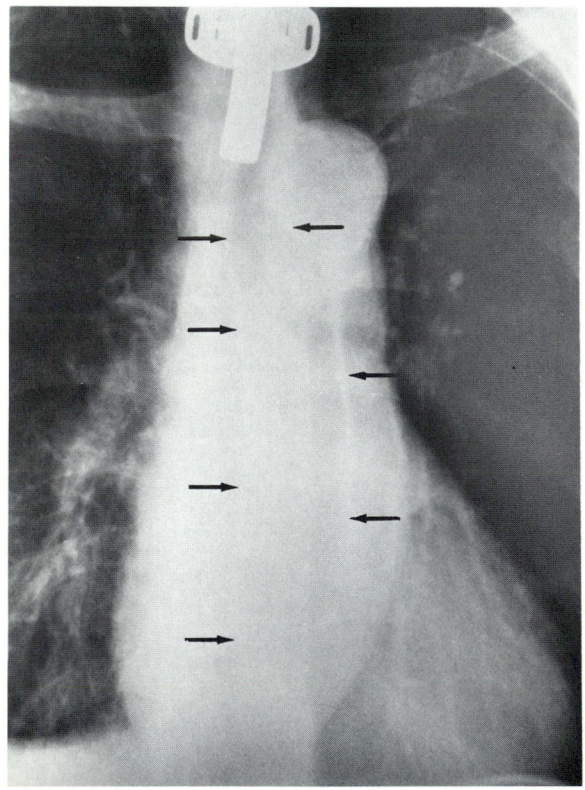

FIG 11–56.—Visualization of the esophageal walls in a postlaryngectomy patient with esophageal speech.

FIG 11–57.—Presbyesophagus. Tertiary contractions ("curling") of the esophagus are frequently found in the elderly and are not usually of significance. (Ref: Zboralske FF, et al: Presbyesophagus: Cineradiographic manifestations. *Radiology* 1964; 82:463.)

FIG 11–58.—An illustration of the great normal distensibility of the infantile esophagus that might be mistaken for megaesophagus.

FIG 11–59.—Transverse striations of the esophagus may be seen as a normal variation, as well as in pathologic states, particularly in association with gastroesophageal reflux. (Refs: Gohel VK, et al: Transverse folds in the human esophagus. *Radiology* 1978; 128:303; and Williams SM, et al: Transverse striations of the esophagus: Association with gastroesophageal reflux. *Radiology* 1983; 146:25.)

FIG 11–60.—The transverse striations seen in **A** are transient, as illustrated in these two films made with the same barium swallow.

FIG 11–61.—Proportional differences in size between the stomach and total abdomen in an infant **(A)** and an adult **(B).** The infant's stomach is proportionately larger, an important concept in avoiding misinterpretation of the size of the air-distended stomach of the infant. (From Keats TE: Pediatric radiology. Some potentially misleading variations from the adult. *Va Med* 1966; 93:630. Used by permission.)

FIG 11–62.—Demonstration of normal degrees of distention of the infantile stomach.

FIG 11–63.—Normal, but marked, gaseous distention of the stomach in a crying infant.

FIG 11–64.—Two examples of the cardioesophageal junction seen en face, simulating a polypoid filling defect in the stomach.

FIG 11–65.—The esophagogastric junction presenting as a polypoid filling defect.

FIG 11–66.—Invagination of the esophageal mucosa at the cardia, simulating a mass lesion. (Ref: de Lorimor AA, Warren JP: Prolapse of the mucosa at the esophagogastric junction. *AJR* 1960; 84:1061.)

FIG 11–67.—The esophageal mucosa, simulating a gastric mass, in a patient with a hiatus hernia. **A,** mucosa is prolapsed into the stomach. **B,** hernia is now present and prolapse is no longer evident. (Ref: Aldridge NH: Transmigration of the lower esophageal mucosa. *Radiology* 1962; 79:962.)

FIG 11–68.—Prolapse of the esophageal mucosa into the stomach (proved at surgery).

FIG 11–69.—Gastric diverticulum in its typical location in the cardia of the stomach.

FIG 11–70.—An additional example of a classic gastric diverticulum.

FIG 11–71.—The left lobe of the liver presenting into the gastric air bubble (proved at surgery), simulating a neoplasm (see Fig 11–28).

FIG 11–72.—Gastric impressions of the left lobe of the liver.

FIG 11–73.—The spleen encroaching on the stomach gas bubble.

FIG 11–74.—Two examples of developmental gastric diverticulum in its classic position.

FIG 11–75.—The impression of a horizontally oriented spleen, simulating a gastric mass.

FIG 11–76 (below).—Splenic impression on the fundus of the stomach. **A,** plain film. **B,** CT confirmation.

FIG 11–77.—Impression of a normal spleen on the stomach. **A,** anteroposterior projection. **B,** left posterior oblique projection. **C,** CT shows the anterior tip of the spleen projecting into the stomach gas bubble.

FIG 11–78.—Normal impressions of the pancreas on the posterior wall of the stomach in an 8-year-old girl. **A,** supine lateral projection; **B,** upright lateral projection.

FIG 11–79.—The impression of the costal margin on the stomach, simulating a mass lesion. **A,** partially filled stomach. **B,** completely filled stomach. (The impression is not as well seen here.)

FIG 11–80.—Additional examples of the impression of the costal margin, simulating a mass lesion.

FIG 11–81.—Barium in the minute folds of the gastric mucosa (confirmed by gastroscopic examination), simulating small ulcers. This entity may also be seen in the colon (see Fig 11–163). **A,** conventional film. **B,** enlargement. (Ref: Stone DD, Keats TE: Anatomical and physiological characteristics of the État Mammelonné, a normal variant of the gastric mucosa. *Radiology* 1973; 107:537.)

FIG 11–82.—The normal appearance of the areae gastricae.

FIG 11–83.—The normal gastric mucosal pattern of the stomach by double contrast examination.

FIG 11–84.—Air bubbles in the stomach, simulating polypoid lesions.

FIG 11–85.—Two examples of artifactual gastric erosions produced by particles of barium. Note the absence of surrounding halos. (Refs: Gohel VK, et al: Double contrast artifacts. *Gastrointest Radiol* 1978; 3:139; Aronchick J, et al: Barium stalactites: Observations on their nature and significance. *Radiology* 1983; 149:588; and Samuel E: Radiology of normal and abnormal gastric mucus. *Br J Radiol* 1987; 60:987.)

FIG 11–86.—Compression films of the stomach, producing "kissing" artifacts simulating mass lesions.

FIG 11–87.—Barium dripping, simulating a gastric diverticulum. (Ref: Shackelford GD: Barium collections in the stomach mimicking intramural diverticula *AJR* 1982; 139:805.)

FIG 11–88.—Normal transverse mucosal folds in the gastric antrum. (Ref: Cho KC, et al: Multiple transverse folds in the gastric antrum. *Radiology* 1987; 164:339.)

FIG 11–89.—Pseudoulceration of the antrum, produced by peristaltic waves seen in **A** and **B,** but not in **C.**

FIG 11–90.—Pseudoulceration of the lesser curve of the antrum produced by peristaltic waves. (Ref: Peavy PW, et al: Gastric pseudo-ulcers: Membrana angularis and pyloric torus defects. *Radiology* 1975; 114:591.)

FIG 11–91.—Additional examples of pseudoulceration of the antrum seen in **A,** but not in **B.** (Ref: Bremner CG: The lesser curve pyloric niche. *Br J Radiol* 1968; 41:291.)

FIG 11–92.—Well-defined muscle band in the body of the stomach.

FIG 11–93.—Functional and transient peristaltic events of the gastric antrum should not be mistaken for mucosal diaphragms. (Ref: Ghahremani GG: Nonobstructive mucosal diaphragms or rings of the gastric antrum in adults. *AJR* 1974; 121:236.)

FIG 11–94.—Additional examples of simulated antral diaphragms. This entity may be particularly confusing in infants. (Ref: Fujioka M, et al: Pseudoweb of the gastric antrum in infants. *Pediatr Radiol* 1980; 9:73.)

FIG 11–95.—Partial gastric diverticulum that could be mistaken for a penetrating ulcer. (Ref: Treichel J, et al: Diagnosis of partial gastric diverticula. *Radiology* 1976; 119:13.)

FIG 11–96.—An additional example of a partial gastric diverticulum.

FIG 11–97.— Additional example of a partial gastric diverticulum.

FIG 11–98.—**A,** transient antral spasm may simulate hypertrophic pyloric stenosis. **B,** film made later in same session shows absence of antral narrowing.

FIG 11–99.—A, impression on greater curvature of the stomach, which simulates pancreatic enlargement. **B,** the impression on the stomach is produced by the filled colon.

FIG 11–100.—*Left,* aberrant pancreas in the antrum. *Right,* aberrant pancreas in the same position showing branching ductal pattern. (From Stone DD, et al: An unusual case of aberrant pancreas in the stomach. *AJR* 1971; 113:125. Used by permission.)

FIG 11–101.—The pyloric canal seen en face, simulating an ulcer.

FIG 11–103.—The air-filled duodenal bulb projected on the gastric antrum, simulating a polyp. Also note air bubbles in the stomach, which might be mistaken for polyps.

FIG 11–102.—An additional example of the pyloric canal ("pyloric star") seen on end, simulating an ulcer.

FIG 11–104.—Prolapse of the antral mucosa into the base of the duodenal bulb. This entity is not usually of clinical significance.

FIG 11–105.— Food (spaghetti) in the duodenal bulb simulating an ascaris.

FIG 11–106.—Brunner's gland hypertrophy may be seen in dyspeptic patients as well as in asymptomatic individuals and should not be mistaken for polyps. (Ref: Fraser GM, et al: Coarse duodenal mucosal folds in patients with dyspepsia and a high gastric acid output. *Clin Radiol* 1971; 22:78.)

FIG 11–107.—Aberrant pancreatic rest in the base of the duodenal bulb.

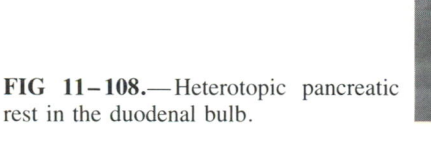

FIG 11–108.—Heterotopic pancreatic rest in the duodenal bulb.

FIG 11–109.—Two examples of inversion of the duodenum (duodenum inversum), a clinically unimportant variation in the course of the duodenal loop that does not connote malrotation. (Ref: Faegenburg O, Bosniak M: Duodenal anomalies in the adult. *AJR* 1962; 88:642.)

FIG 11–110.—Spot films to show normal, but prominent, mucosal folds of the duodenal bulb. Note pliability and changing pattern.

FIG 11–111.—The lumen of the second portion of the duodenum seen en face, simulating an intraluminal lesion.

FIG 11–112.—A, the lumen of the second portion of the duodenum seen on end, simulating a filling defect. **B,** the pseudolesion is not seen on subsequent film.

FIG 11–113.—A, air bubbles in the duodenal bulb, simulating polypoid filling defects. **B,** normal appearance seen on repeat examination.

FIG 11–114.—Two examples of circular mucosal filling defects said to be due to ectopic gastric mucosa. (Ref: Smithuis RHM, Vos CG: Heterotopic gastric mucosa in the duodenal bulb: Relationship to peptic ulcer. *AJR* 1989; 152:59.) Benign lymphoid hyperplasia may also produce similar filling defects (Ref: Govoni AF: Benign lymphoid hyperplasia of the duodenal bulb. *Gastrointest Radiol* 1976; 1:267.)

FIG 11–115.—A, simulated "bull's-eye" lesion in the duodenum in a patient with melanoma originally diagnosed as a metastatic deposit. This is produced by the lumen of the second portion of the duodenum, not seen in **B.**

FIG 11–116.—Other examples of air bubbles in the duodenal bulb, simulating filling defects.

FIG 11–117.—Simulated ulcer at the apex of the bulb due to peristaltic contraction. (Ref: Burrell M, Toffler R: Flexural pseudolesions of the duodenum. *Radiology* 1976; 120:313.)

FIG 11–118.—Four examples of flexural pseudo-masses or ulcers at the apex of the bulb due to prominence of the mucosal folds. (Ref: Nelson JA, et al: Duodenal pseudopolyp—the flexure fallacy. *AJR* 1975; 123:262.)

FIG 11–119.—Impression of the common duct in a normal 18-year-old woman.

FIG 11–120.—A, impressions of the gallbladder on the superior aspect of the duodenum (←) and the antrum of the stomach (←). **B,** cholecystogram shows position of the gallbladder in reference to the impressions in **B.**
(Ref: Smeets R, Op Den Orth JO: Gallbladder: Common cause of antral pad sign. *AJR* 1979; 132:571.)

FIG 11–121.—The ampulla of Vater in normal subjects. **A,** 2-week-old infant. **B,** adult.

FIG 11–122.—Apparent widening of the duodenal loop produced by high position of the transverse colon, which elevates the stomach and uncovers more of the duodenal loop than is normally seen.

FIG 11–123.—Medial displacement of the second portion of the duodenum by the right kidney. (Ref: Yoong P, House R: Deceptive duodenal deformity. *Br J Radiol* 1980; 53:1012.)

FIG 11–124.—Normal prominence of the pattern of the valvulae conniventes of the small bowel in a 2-year-old boy.

FIG 11–125.—Normal grouping of the proximal loops of the jejunum of the left midabdomen, not to be confused with an internal hernia.

FIG 11–126.—Two examples of malrotation of the bowel with ramification of the proximal small bowel on the right, rather than on the left (as in Fig 11–125).

FIG 11–127.—Abnormal pattern of the duodenum and proximal small bowel due to large amount of mucus in the stomach.

FIG 11–128.—Three examples of unusual small bowel patterns in infants due to mucus-impregnated barium.

FIG 11–129.—Normal prominent mucosal patterns of the small bowel of young children. **A,** 2-year-old. **B,** 3-year-old.

FIG 11–130.—Normal mucosal pattern of the adult small bowel by double contrast examination.

FIG 11–131.—Areas of peristaltic contraction may be mistaken for ascariasis in children (see Fig 11–136).

FIG 11–132.—Unusual small bowel pattern resulting from large amount of fat in the mesentery.

FIG 11–133.—The "cobblestone" terminal ileum in a 3-year-old boy. This normal variation is due to the large amounts of lymphoid tissue in this portion of the bowel and should not be mistaken for evidence of inflammatory bowel disease. (Ref: Lassrich MA: Nonspecific changes in the terminal ileum of children. *Fortschr Roentgenstr* 1961; 95:757.)

FIG 11–134.—Normal lymphoid hyperplasia of the terminal ileum in a 16-year-old-boy, a further reflection of the process illustrated in Figure 11–133. These changes are often misinterpreted as evidence of Crohn's disease.

FIG 11–135.—Lymphoid hyperplasia in the terminal ileum in a healthy 62-year-old man.

FIG 11–136.—Mucosal folds in the terminal ileum simulating ascaris.

FIG 11–137.—A, distended uninary bladder in a young child, displacing the small bowel and colon. **B,** disappearance of displacement after catheterization and removal of 300 mL of urine (see Fig 11–144).

FIG 11–138.—Proportional difference in the size of the colon and the abdomen in a 3-year-old child (**A**) and an adult (**B**). The colon of the infant, as well as that of the child, occupies a proportionately larger area of the abdomen and its size should not be mistaken for megacolon. (From Keats TE: Pediatric radiology: Some potentially misleading variations from the adult. *Va Med* 1966; 93:630. Used by permission.)

FIG 11–139.—An illustration of the great distensibility of the normal juvenile colon in a 2½-year-old child.

FIG 11–140.—Malrotation of the bowel. The colon lies entirely in the left side of the abdomen. The *arrows* indicate the ascending colon.

FIG 11–141.—"Overrotation" of the colon, with an elongated ascending portion and the cecum presenting in the midabdomen *(arrow)*.

FIG 11–142.—Mobile cecum. Note the change of position following evacuation (B). While not clinically significant in itself, such mobility predisposes to volvulus.

FIG 11–143 (left).—Subhepatic cecum (←) and appendix (⊬).

FIG 11–144 (right).—Displacement of the colon and small bowel by a distended urinary bladder in a 5-year-old boy.

FIG 11–145 (below).—Lateral displacement of the right kidney by the colon. *Left*, plain film tomogram from an intravenous urogram. *Right*, CT scan shows the lateral displacement of the kidney by the ascending colon. (From Silverman PM, et al: Lateral displacement of the right kidney by the colon: An anatomic variation demonstrated by CT. *AJR* 1983; 140:313. Used by permission.)

FIG 11–146.—Pressure on the superior aspect of the hepatic flexure produced by the liver edge.

FIG 11–147.—Pressure defect on the proximal descending colon produced by the spleen.

FIG 11–148.—Simulated mass in the descending colon produced by the spinous process of the adjacent lumbar vertebra.

FIG 11–149.—Four examples of large ileocecal valves that simulate polypoid masses.

FIG 11–150.—Retrograde prolapse of the ileocecal valve, simulating a neoplasm of the terminal ileum. **A,** before prolapse. **B,** after prolapse. (From Hatten HP Jr, et al: Retrograde prolapse of the ileocecal valve. *AJR* 1977; 128:755. Used by permission.)

FIG 11–151.—Mobile cecum with the ileocecal valve entering from the right side.

FIG 11–152.—*Top left*, intussusception of the base of the normal appendix on low pressure barium enema *(arrow)*. *Top right*, partial reduction and filling of the appendix with medium pressure. *Bottom*, complete reduction with high pressure. Note small filling defects in the cecal mucosa in the *top right* and *bottom* figures representing lymphoid follicles.

FIG 11–153.—Prominent, but normal, haustral pattern in a healthy 40-year-old man. Note simulation of diverticula. **A,** preevacuation. **B,** postevacuation.

FIG 11–154.—Paucity of haustral markings in the left half of the colon is not uncommon in normal individuals and those with prolonged cathartic abuse. This appearance may simulate that of chronic ulcerative colitis. **A,** preevacuation. **B,** postevacuation. (Ref: Plum GE, et al: Prolonged cathartic abuse resulting in roentgen evidence suggestive of enterocolitis. *AJR* 1960; 83:919.)

FIG 11–155.—The colon by double contrast with a pattern that simulates small bowel, probably the result of barium in the innominate grooves.

FIG 11–156.—A, physiologic colonic sphincter, simulating colonic neoplasm. B, the alteration is not seen in the postevacuation film. (Ref: Templeton A: Colon sphincters simulating organic disease. *Radiology* 1960; 75:237.)

FIG 11–157.—A, an additional example of a physiologic sphincter, simulating a neoplasm, not seen in the follow-up examination (B). (Ref: Cimmino CV: Roentgen-diagnostic value of spasm of certain colonic "sphincters." *Va Med* 1965; 92:317.)

FIG 11–158.—Two examples of a physiologic sphincter closely resembling an annular carcinoma.

FIG 11–159.—Elongation, elevation, and narrowing of the pelvic colon secondary to fat accumulation in the pelvis. This entity should not be confused with the changes due to pelvic neoplasm. The bladder is similarly altered (see Fig 13–78) (Ref: Fogg LB, Smyth JW: Pelvic lipomatosis: A condition simulating pelvic neoplasm. *Radiology* 1968; 90:558.)

FIG 11–160.—An additional example of the colonic changes in pelvic lipomatosis.

FIG 11–161.—Pre- and postevacuation films showing displacement of the sigmoid colon by the iliopsoas muscle. A similar defect may be seen in the ascending colon and the terminal ileum in some patients. (Refs: Martel W: Displacement of the intestine by the iliopsoas muscle. *AJR* 1965; 94:399; and Duprat G Jr, et al: Bowel displacement due to psoas muscle hypertrophy. *J Can Assoc Radiol* 1983; 34:64.)

FIG 11–162.—Pre- and postevacuation films of the rectum in lateral projection, showing increase in the retrorectal space due to obesity and not to interposed pathology. This may also be seen in Cushing's disease. (Refs: Fennessy JJ, et al: Early roentgen manifestations of mild ulcerative colitis and proctitis. *Radiology* 1966; 87:848; and Yagan R, Marmslya G: Increased retrorectal space on barium enema in pelvic lipomatosis. *Appl Radiol* April 1988, vol 17, p 36.)

FIG 11–163.—Barium in the innominate folds of the hepatic flexure, simulating mucosal ulceration. **A,** preevacuation film does not demonstrate the folds. **B,** postevacuation film nicely shows the barium in the folds. (Ref: Williams I: Innominate grooves in the surface of mucosa. *Radiology* 1965; 84:877.)

FIG 11–164.—Two examples of the innominate grooves of the colon. These can be distinguished from ulcerations by their inconsistency. (Refs: Frank DF, et al: Pseudoulcerations of the colon on barium examination. *Gastrointest Radiol* 1977; 2:129; and Cole FM: Innominate grooves of the colon: Morphological characteristics and etiologic mechanisms. *Radiology* 1978; 128:41.)

FIG 11–165.—Lymphoid follicles in healthy children. **A,** 3-year-old. **B,** 13-year-old. These lesions are not believed to be of significance but may be confused with polyposis coli. (Ref: Laufer I, deSa D: Lymphoid follicular pattern: A normal feature of the pediatric colon. *AJR* 1978; 130:51.)

FIG 11–166.—Two examples of lymphoid follicles of the colon in adults, a finding of no clinical significance per se. **A,** 63-year-old man. **B,** 43-year old man. (Ref: Kelvin FM, et al: Lymphoid follicular pattern of the colon in adults. *AJR* 1979; 133:821.)

FIG 11–167.—Fat droplets in the colon after castor oil ingestion, simulating polypoid lesions.

FIG 11–168.—"Rectal ears" in a 1-month-old baby. These are transitory protrusions of the rectum into the inguinal rings. (Ref: Kassner EG, et al: "Rectal ears." *J Can Assoc Radiol* 1975; 26:125.)

FIG 11–169.—Pressure effect of a full bladder on the sigmoid colon. **A** and **B,** full bladder. **C** and **D,** after bladder is emptied. (Ref: Kleinhaus V, Kaftori J: Rectosigmoid pseudostenosis due to urinary retention. *Radiology* 1978; 127:645.)

FIG 11–170.—Another example of the effect of a distended urinary bladder on the rectosigmoid colon.

FIG 11–171.—Two examples of the impressions of the levator ani muscles on the rectum in children.

FIG 11–172.—Two examples of "kissing" artifacts produced by contrast of the rectal balloon and the rectal wall. (Ref: Gohel VK, et al: Double contrast artifacts. *Gastrointest Radiol* 1978; 3:139.)

FIG 11–173.—A, "kissing" artifacts of the rectum produced by balloon contact. **B,** after removal of balloon.

FIG 11–174.—Two examples of alterations seen in double contrast examinations due to strands of mucus, not to be confused with linear ulceration.

FIG 11–175.—Two examples of sacral foramina projecting through the colon, simulating filling defects.

FIG 11–176.—Leakage of barium into the vagina during barium enema simulates extravasation due to rupture of the rectum.

FIG 11–177.—Pelvic phleboliths, simulating colonic diverticula, on barium enema.

FIG 11–178.—Differences in proportion in the size of the liver and the total abdominal area in the child (**A**) and adult (**B**). The child's liver occupies a proportionately larger portion of the abdomen. (From Keats TE: Pediatric radiology. Some potentially misleading variations from the adult. *Va Med* 1966; 93:630. Used by permission.)

FIG 11–179.—Riedel's lobe of the liver, simulating an abdominal mass. (Ref: Reitemeier HR, et al: Riedel's lobe of the liver. *Gastroenterology* 1958; 34:1090.)

FIG 11–180.—Additional examples of Riedel's lobe.

FIG 11–181.—Intrahepatic gallbladder.

FIG 11–182.—Intermittent herniation of the gallbladder into the lesser sac. **A,** normal position. **B** and **C,** herniated position.

FIG 11–183.—Gallbladder variations; incomplete septation of the distal end. (Ref: Rabinovitch J, et al: Congenital anomalies of the gallbladder. *Ann Surg* 1958; 148:161.)

FIG 11–184.—Three examples of complete compartmentalization of the distal end of the gallbladder.

FIG 11–185.—**A,** double gallbladder (proved). **B,** partial duplication. **C,** flexion of a long gallbladder, simulating duplication. (Ref: Guyer PB, et al: Congenital double gallbladder. A review and report of two cases. *Br J Radiol* 1967; 40:214.)

FIG 11–186.—Gallbladder variations. **A,** an elongated tortuous gallbladder. **B** and **C,** flexion of the distal end of the gallbladder.

FIG 11–187.—Two examples of gallbladders with multiple septa.

FIG 11–188.—Halo of radiolucency around the gallbladder due to fat, not to be confused with emphysematous cholecystitis.

FIG 11–189.—**A,** phrygian cap, simulating a calculus. **B,** true nature of the density is demonstrated on steep left posterior oblique projection.

FIG 11–190.—A, the neck of the gallbladder seen en face, simulating a calculus. **B,** in the oblique projection, the neck of the gallbladder is demonstrated.

FIG 11–191.—A, precipitation of contrast medium into the gallbladder, simulating biliary calculi. **B,** repeat cholecystogram 3 days later is normal. (Ref: Theander G: Pseudoconcretions in precipitate of contrast medium in the gallbladder. *AJR* 1960; 83:828.)

FIG 11–192.—Stratification of opacified bile in oral cholecystography. This has no significance in itself. (Ref: Lindenbraten LD: The layering phenomenon of the gallbladder and the roentgen diagnosis of cholecystitis. *ROFO* 1971; 115:457.)

FIG 11–193.—A, stratification of bile with the patient in the horizontal position, producing edge-ring effect that might be mistaken for a large calculus. **B,** same examination after adequate mixing of bile and contrast medium. (Ref: Wright JT: Stratification of bile. *Australas Radiol* 1973; 17:157.)

FIG 11–194.—A, simulated gallstones due to inadequate mixing of bile and contrast material. **B,** normal appearance after adequate mixing.

FIG 11–195.—A and **B,** layering phenomenon in intravenous cholangiography is also without clinical significance. (Ref: Twigg HL, Zelna A: Stratification in intravenous cholangiography. *Radiology* 1963; 80:774.)

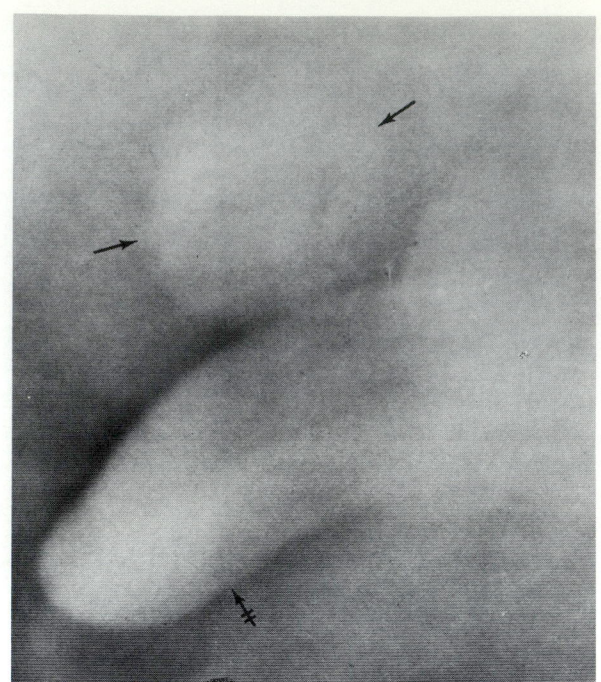

FIG 11–196.—Fluid in the duodenal bulb (←), simulating duplication of the gallbladder, which is seen below (⫲).

FIG 11–197.—**A,** prone film—apparent "reformed gallbladder" seen on intravenous cholangiogram after cholecystectomy and produced by contrast material in the duodenal bulb and gastric antrum. **B,** supine film—gas has replaced the contrast material.

FIG 11–198.—**A,** intravenous cholangiogram shows what appears to be a gallbladder with a large, faceted stone within. **B,** later film shows the true gallbladder (→) and indicates that the image in **A** is the duodenal bulb filled with contrast material (↠) with the outline of the pylorus within.

FIG 11–199.—The normal common duct visualized tomographically by virtue of its surrounding periductal fat. (Ref: Shaub MS, et al: Peribiliary fat. *AJR* 1975; 123:330.) This entity may be confused with pneumobilia. (Ref: Govani AF, Meyers MA: Pseudopneumobilia. *Radiology* 1976; 118:526.)

FIG 11–200.—Three examples of the pylorus of the stomach, simulating a fissured biliary calculus. In **B** and **C** the air in the duodenal bulb simulates emphysematous cholecystitis with stone.

FIG 11–201.—Calcified costal cartilage, which simulates biliary calculi.

FIG 11–202.—Accessory hepatic duct entering low in the common duct.

FIG 11–203.—Accessory right hepatic duct.

FIG 11–204.—Intramural cystic duct remnant. This portion of the cystic duct lies within the wall of the common duct and is not detectable at cholecystectomy.

FIG 11–205.—*Left,* pseudocalculus sign seen in cholangiography is produced by muscular contraction of the distal end of the duct and should not be mistaken for a calculus. *Right,* second film in the same examination does not show the defect. (Ref: Mujahed Z, Evans JA: Pseudocalculus defect in cholangiography. *AJR* 1972; 116:337.) The same defect may be seen on intravenous cholangiography. (Ref: Martinez LO, Cohen G: The pseudocalculus sign in intravenous cholangiography. *South Med J* 1972; 65:1066.)

FIG 11–206.—A, the pseudocalculus sign in a dilated biliary tree. B, normal appearance after contraction has been relieved.

FIG 11–207.—The pseudocalculus sign, with a small amount of contrast material in the duct, simulating a stone.

FIG 11–208.—Low insertion of the cystic duct (←) resulting in a very short common duct (⇤).

FIG 11–209.—A, contrast and food in the duodenal bulb simulates a gallbladder with stones on cholangiography. B, after peristalsis has cleared the duodenum.

FIG 11–211.—Two examples of the accessory duct of Santorini arising from the duct of Wirsung.

FIG 11–210.—Duplication of the distal end of the pancreatic duct shown by endoscopic retrograde cholangiopancreatography.

FIG 11–212.—Costal cartilage mistaken for the right hepatic duct with stones.

912   *The Soft Tissues of the Abdomen—The Liver and Biliary Tract*

Chapter 12

The Soft Tissues of the Pelvis

Pages
915 to **921**

Figures
12–1 to **12–23**

FIG 12–1.—Circular areas of radiolucency due to fat in the buttocks.

FIG 12–2.—The shadows of the levator ani muscles (←). The obturator internus muscles are also seen (⫟). (Ref: Levene G, Kaufman JA: The diagnostic significance of roentgenologic soft tissue shadows in the pelvis. *AJR* 1958; 79:697.)

FIG 12–3.—Contraction of the levator ani muscles will produce evanescent shadows in the pelvis in a given patient. **A,** levator ani muscles not seen. **B,** same patient with muscle contractions, showing intrusion of the bladder outline.

FIG 12–4.—Stripes of radiolucency due to fat accumulations between the muscle bundles of the gluteus maximus.

FIG 12–5.—The shadow of the uterus seen indenting the superior aspect of the urinary bladder.

FIG 12–6.—Unusual configuration of pelvic phleboliths, elongated on the patient's right (←) and bifid on the left (⊬).

FIG 12–7.—The sigmoid colon simulating a pelvic mass.

FIG 12–8.—Calcified epiploic appendages, which have fallen into the pelvis, will shift from side to side as illustrated in this patient. (Refs: Holt JF, MacIntyre RS: Calcified omental fat deposits: Their roentgenologic significance. *AJR* 1948; 60:612; and Borg SA, et al: A mobile calcified amputated appendix epiploica. *AJR* 1976; 127:349.)

FIG 12–9.—Examples of calcification in Cooper's ligament. This is seen in the elderly as an unusual form of physiologic calcification. (Ref: Steinfeld, JR, et al: Calcification in Cooper's ligament. *AJR* 1974; 121:107.)

FIG 12–10.—**A** and **B,** examples of calcification of the sacrospinous ligaments.

FIG 12–11.—Calcification in the anterior sacral ligament (→) and in the sacrotuberous ligament (↠).

FIG 12–12.—Calcification of the sacrotuberous ligaments. **A,** frontal projection. **B,** lateral projection.

FIG 12–13.—Long linear calcification of the left sacrotuberous ligament.

FIG 12–14.—Calcification in the piriform muscles in an 82-year-old woman.

FIG 12–15.—Calcification, probably within the coccygoanal ligament.

FIG 12–16.—Calcification in the inferior pubic ligaments.

FIG 12–17.—Ossification of the obturator foramen. (Ref: Birkner R, Consentius K: Ossification of the obturator foramen. *ROFO* 1977; 127:72.)

FIG 12–18.—Multiple pelvic phleboliths of varying sizes.

FIG 12–19.—Phlebolith in the spermatic cord.

FIG 12–20.—Vulvar phleboliths.

FIG 12–21.—Calcification in the uterine arteries in an elderly woman.

FIG 12–22.—Calcification of the fallopian tubes in an elderly woman.

FIG 12–23.—Two examples of calcified seminal vesicles. *Left*, 50-year-old man. *Right*, 71-year-old man.

Chapter 13

The Genitourinary Tract

FIG 13–1.—Apparent absence of one psoas muscle. This is seen in many normal individuals and is not necessarily of significance. (Ref: Elkin M, Cohen G: Diagnostic value of psoas shadow. *Clin Radiol* 1962; 13:210.)

FIG 13–2.—The low-lying left kidney. The left kidney lies at a level lower than the right in 5% of normal individuals. This finding is not therefore necessarily indicative of displacement. (Ref: McClelland RE: A low-lying left kidney. *J Urol* 1956; 75:198.)

FIG 13–3.—Costophrenic sulcus and the edge of the lung producing unusual appearance in the nephrogram of the right kidney.

FIG 13–4.—The splenic impression (←) on the left kidney that produces a "bump" in its midportion (↤). (Ref: Olutola PO, et al: Unusual renal distortion and displacement due to the spleen. *Pediatr Radiol* 1982; 12:185.)

FIG 13–5.—The hepatic impression (←) on the right kidney that produces a "bump" in its midportion (⊬). **A,** urogram. **B,** angiogram. (Ref: Doppman JL, Shapiro R: Some normal renal variants. *AJR* 1964; 92:1380.)

FIG 13–6.—Fetal lobulation of the kidneys.

FIG 13–7.—Nonsignificant variation in outline of the right kidney.

FIG 13–8.—Two examples of the dromedary left kidney, an anatomic variation that simulates a mass lesion. (Ref: Harrow BP, Sloane JA: The dromedary left kidney. *AJR* 1962; 88:148.)

FIG 13–9.—The gastric fundus, simulating a suprarenal mass. **A,** before ingestion of barium. **B,** after ingestion of barium. (Ref: Martire JR, Goldman SM: Left suprarenal pseudotumor. *Radiobiologiia* 1977; 17:12.) This pseudotumor may opacify on angiography and further obscure its proper identification. (Ref: Bjorn-Hansen RW, O'Brien DS: Aortographic opacification of the gastric fundus simulating neoplasm. *AJR* 1967; 100:408.)

FIG 13–10.—Two examples of spurious suprarenal masses produced by the duodenal bulb. Fluid and air filled *(left);* fluid filled *(right).*

FIG 13–11.—Two examples of renal pseudotumors produced by the spleen. (Ref: Madayag M, et al: Renal and suprarenal pseudotumors caused by variations of the spleen. *Radiology* 1972; 105:43.)

FIG 13–12.—Pelvic kidney.

FIG 13–13.—Ptotic right kidney. Note the configuration of its collecting system and its position in the lateral projection.

FIG 13–14.—Variations in renal outline of the right kidney with respiration. **A,** expiration. **B,** inspiration.

9 yrs
ago

R L
13.5 / 13.8

R L
11.5 / 13.8

FIG 13–15.—Anterior displacement and rotation of the kidneys by retroperitoneal fat. **A,** year 1—normal appearance of kidneys. **B,** year 9—the contour of the right kidney has altered and appears shorter in its vertical dimensions. **C,** CT shows anterior displacement of the right kidney by fat. (Ref: Hooge WA, et al: Anterior displacement of kidneys by fat. *J Can Assoc Radiol* 1980; 31:143.)

FIG 13–16.—Duplication variant producing discrepancy in renal size. The left kidney is duplex and is distinctly larger than the right. **A,** plain film. **B,** urogram.

FIG 13–17.—**A,** costal cartilage calcification, simulating renal calculi. **B,** the calcification is obscured by the contrast material in the urogram.

FIG 13–18.—Multiplicity of calyces. This is an atavistic variant that may be mistaken for a pathologic state.

FIG 13–19.—The unicalyx kidney. Another atavistic variant, representing the normal arrangement in monkeys, dogs, and rabbits. (Ref: Harrison RB, et al: A solitary calyx in a human kidney. *Radiology* 1976; 121:310.)

FIG 13–20 (left).—Megacalyces of the left kidney. This variant is often unilateral and represents a malformation of the renal papillae. The cortex is normal, but the medulla is hypoplastic. The dilated calyces and reduced parenchymal thickness resemble obstructive hydronephrosis or postobstructive atrophy. (Ref: Talner LB, Gittes RF: Megacalyces: Further observations and differentiation from obstructive renal disease. *AJR* 1974; 121:473.)

FIG 13–21.—**A,** megacalyces of the right kidney. **B,** detailed view of right kidney.

FIG 13–22.—Bilateral megacalyces. This condition may be genetically transmitted. (Ref: Lam AH: Familial megacalyces with autosomal recessive inheritance. *Pediatr Radiol* 1988; 19:28.)

FIG 13–23.—Two examples of extrarenal collecting systems. The claw-like configuration of the infundibula, best seen in the right kidney in **A,** is characteristic of this variation in development. Fifty percent of these individuals have associated renal disease. **B,** bilateral extrarenal collecting systems. (Ref: Malament M, et al: Extrarenal calyces: Their relationship to renal disease. *AJR* 1961; 86:823.)

FIG 13–24.—Miniature calyx. Tubular blush, produced by contrast material in the collecting tubules, is seen as a halo around this calyx. (Ref: Kunin M: The abortive calix: Variation in appearance and differential diagnosis. *AJR* 1982; 139:931.)

FIG 13–25.—Accessory calyx arising from the middle calyceal group.

FIG 13–26.—Small calyceal diverticulum.

FIG 13–27.—Calyceal diverticulum. *Left*, early filling. *Right*, late filling.

FIG 13–28.—Calyx seen on end, simulating a filling defect.

FIG 13–29.—An aberrant renal papilla entering the infundibulum of the lower pole. (Ref: Binder R, et al: Aberrant papillae and other filling defects of the renal pelvis. *AJR* 1972; 114:746.)

FIG 13–30.—Aberrant renal papilla entering the renal pelvis. This variant may be associated with hematuria.

FIG 13–31.—Another example of an aberrant renal papilla entering the renal pelvis.

FIG 13–32.—Flat upper pole calyceal groups that might be mistaken for distortion by adjacent mass.

FIG 13–33.—Large composite upper pole calyceal groups.

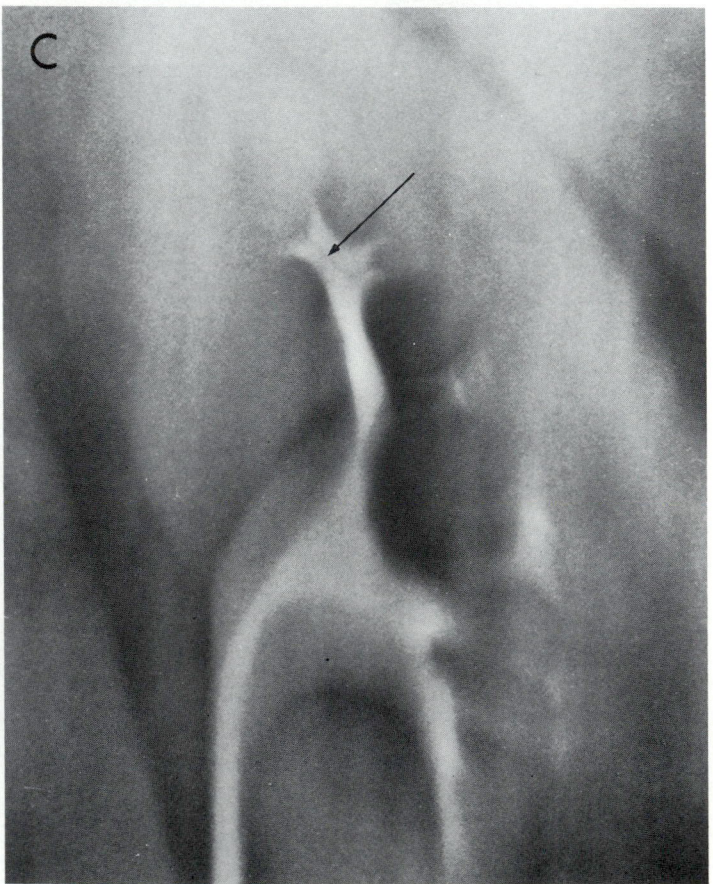

FIG 13–34.—**A** and **B,** mucosal folds seen within calyces and infundibula. **C,** tomogram of left kidney shows the folds in the superior calyx. These folds do not indicate abnormality.

FIG 13–35.—A, incomplete filling of the calyces and infundibula may simulate a mass lesion. **B,** mass effect is no longer seen with adequate filling.

FIG 13–36.—Bulge in the suprahilar region of the right kidney representing the hilar lip or renal uncus. **A,** plain film. **B,** nephrotomogram. (Ref: Feldman AE, et al: Renal pseudotumors: An anatomic-radiologic classification. *J Urol* 1978; 120:133.)

FIG 13–37.—Deformity of the collecting system due to excessive invagination of the cortical tissue in forming Bertin's columns. This entity is often found in cases with duplications of the collecting system and may simulate a neoplasm. The diagnosis is made by arteriography. **A,** plain film. **B,** arteriogram. **C,** nephrogram. (Ref: Lopez FA: Renal pseudotumors. *AJR* 1970; 109:172.)

FIG 13–38.—**A,** an additional example of the deformity of the collecting system due to Bertin's columns. **B,** nephrogram.

FIG 13–39.—Renal pelvic lipomatosis. The deposition of large amounts of normal fat in the renal pelvis produces radiolucency, stretching, and elongation of the infundibula, best seen in the right kidney (←). On occasion, it may resemble the changes of polycystic disease as seen in the left kidney (⇐). (Ref: Ambos MA, et al: Replacement lipomatosis of the kidney. *AJR* 1978; 130:1087.)

FIG 13–40.—Backflow. **A,** pyelovenous. **B,** pyelolymphatic. **C,** pyelotubular. **D,** tubular blush produced by contrast material in the collecting tubules of the renal papillae. This should not be mistaken for the tubular ectasia of the medullary sponge kidney. (Ref: Ohlson L: Normal collecting ducts: Visualization at urography. *Radiology* 1989; 170:33.)

FIG 13–41.—Accessory renal hilus. *Left,* nephrogram shows a defect in the superior pole of the kidney *(arrow). Right,* renal angiogram shows a renal artery entering the kidney at the area of the defect. A separate renal artery supplies the remainder of the kidney. Arteriography is usually necessary to distinguish the accessory renal hilus from a pathologic process. (Courtesy of Dr. Thomas F. Stephenson.)

FIG 13–42.—Two examples of vascular impressions on the renal pelvis. Most of these are not clinically important. (Ref: Baum S, Gillenwater JY: Renal artery impressions on renal pelvis. *J Urol* 1966; 95:139.)

FIG 13–43.—Four additional examples of vascular impressions on the collecting systems. (Ref: Nebesar RA, et al: Renal vascular impression: Incidence and clinical significance. *AJR* 1967; 101: 719.)

FIG 13–44.—Tortuous infundibulum.

FIG 13–45.—Unusual bifid collecting system.

FIG 13–46.—An abortive duplication of the renal pelvis.

FIG 13–47.—Two examples of extrarenal pelves that simulate the changes of hydronephrosis. **A,** bilateral extrarenal pelves. **B,** duplicated extrarenal pelvis of the right kidney only.

FIG 13–48.—A, simulated hydronephrosis produced by massive distention of the bladder *(arrows)*. B, appearance after bladder is emptied.

FIG 13–49.—"Yo-yo" effect (saddle reflux) of pelvic emptying in duplex kidneys. A, the upper segment of the right kidney is emptying, and the lower segment filling. B, the lower segment contracts, and the upper segment fills by reflux. These are normal dynamics in duplex kidneys. The transient distention of the upper segment could be misinterpreted as pathologic dilatation. (Ref: Privett JRJ, et al: The incidence and importance of renal duplication. *Clin Radiol* 1976; 27:521.)

FIG 13–50.—"Pigtail" renal pelvis, showing unusual course of the proximal portion of the ureter.

FIG 13–51.—Transverse folds in the proximal ureter represent a normal variation in infants. They are believed to represent a persistence of normal fetal tortuosities. (From Kirks DR, et al: Transverse folds in the proximal ureter: A normal variation in infants. *AJR* 1978; 130:463. Used by permission.)

FIG 13–52.—Normal deviations of the ureter caused by the iliopsoas muscles. (Ref: Levine RB, et al: Ureteral deviation due to iliopsoas hypertrophy. *AJR* 1969; 107:756.)

FIG 13–53.—Peristalsis of the ureters should not be mistaken for pathologic changes.

FIG 13–54.—The retrocaval ureter, coursing around the posterior aspect of the inferior vena cava. (Ref: Emmett JL, Witten DM: *Clinical Urography,* ed 3. Philadelphia, WB Saunders Co, 1971, p 1327.)

FIG 13–55.—Full column filling of the ureters secondary to distention of the urinary bladder.

FIG 13–56.—Variation in position of ureters with technique of exposure. **A,** in the true lateral position, the upper kidney and ureter drop anteriorly. **B,** in the cross-table lateral view, the location of the ureters and kidneys can be compared more accurately. (Ref: Cook IK, et al: Determination of the normal position of the upper urinary tract on the lateral abdominal urogram. *Radiology* 1971; 99:499.)

FIG 13–57.—Effects of respiration on ureteral configuration. **A,** expiration. **B,** inspiration.

FIG 13–58.—Visualization of the left ureter without contrast agent due to periureteral fat.

FIG 13–59.—Medial deviation of the distal ureters as a normal variant due to iliopsoas hypertrophy, and not secondary to retroperitoneal fibrosis. (Ref: Saldino RM, Palubinskas AJ: Medial placement of the ureters: A normal variant which may simulate retroperitoneal fibrosis. *J Urol* 1972; 107:582.)

FIG 13–60.—Ureteral displacement by hypertrophy of the iliopsoas muscles. This is a misleading finding, seen particularly in muscular young men, that may be unilateral. (Ref: Levine RB, et al: Ureteral deviation due to iliopsoas hypertrophy. *AJR* 1969; 107:756.)

FIG 13–61.—**A,** medial deviation of the ureters by hypertrophied iliopsoas muscles. **B,** the muscles also produce medial displacement of the bladder. (Ref: Wechsler RJ, Brennan RE: Teardrop bladder: Additional considerations. *Radiology* 1982; 144:281.)

FIG 13–62.—Two examples of unilateral deviation of the ureter due to unilateral iliopsoas hypertrophy, both proved at laparotomy. (Ref: Ziter FMH: Unilateral ureteral deviation due to iliopsoas muscle hypertrophy. *J Can Assoc Radiol* 1974; 25: 327.)

FIG 13–63.—Deviation of the distal right ureter produced by an ectatic iliac artery in an elderly man.

FIG 13–64.—Three examples of blind duplication of the ureters. **A,** termination at the renal pelvis. **B** and **C,** termination in the pelvis. (Ref: Albers DD, et al: Blind-ending branch of a bifid ureter: Report of three cases. *J Urol* 1968; 99:160.)

FIG 13–65.—**A,** a pseudoectopic ureter seen in the prone position, in which the contrast material in the bladder gravitates toward the head into the dependent anterior dome and leaves the trigone area filled with non-opacified urine. The distal ureters appear to extend below the bladder. **B,** supine film does not show the same effect seen in **A.** (Ref: Riggs W Jr, Seibert J: Pseudoectopic ureter on prone urogram. *Radiology* 1973; 106:391.)

FIG 13–66.—Two examples of the ureteral jet phenomenon. A stream of opaque medium leaving the ureter may simulate an anomalous configuration of the ureter. Note the impaction of the jet on the bladder wall in **A** (→). (Ref: Kalmon EH, et al: Ureteral jet phenomenon. Stream of opaque medium simulating anomalous configuration of ureter. *Radiology* 1955; 65:933.)

FIG 13–67.—Asymmetry of the pelvic ureters in normal females, with medial deviation of the distal right ureter, is a normal variation. (Ref: Kabakian HA, et al: Asymmetry of the pelvic ureters in normal females. *AJR* 1976; 127:723.)

FIG 13–68.—**A,** apparent filling defect in the distal left ureter, resulting from peristalsis. **B,** after peristaltic wave has passed, the impression is no longer seen.

FIG 13–69.—Proportional difference in size between the bladder and the total abdomen in the infant (**A**) and adult (**B**). The bladder in the infant (as well as the child) is capable of a much greater proportional degree of distention. (From Keats TE: Pediatric radiology: Some potentially misleading variations from the adult. *Va Med* 1966; 93:630. Used by permission.)

FIG 13–70.—**A,** normal distention of the bladder in a 2-year-old, displacing the small bowel. **B,** after voiding.

FIG 13–71.—Visualization of the bladder wall as a result of the difference in radiographic density between muscle and urine.

FIG 13–72.—Perivesical fat producing an appearance simulating emphysematous cystitis.

FIG 13–73.—"Bladder ears," a transitory extraperitoneal herniation of the bladder in infants. This is believed to represent a transient variation in normal development. (Ref: Allen RP, Condon VR: Transitory extraperitoneal hernia of the bladder in infants. *Radiology* 1961; 77:979.)

FIG 13–74.—Examples of unilateral "bladder ears."

FIG 13–75.—"Bladder ears" in a 53-year-old woman due to laxity of the inguinal rings.

FIG 13–76.—The uterine impression on the bladder. **A**, the shadow of the uterus is seen indenting the bladder. **B**, the shadow of the uterus is not seen above the impression on the bladder.

FIG 13–77.—Normal physiologic variations in contour of the base of the bladder during voiding. Note the asymmetric urethral distention in **A** (→) and the indentation produced posteriorly by the trigonal plate in **B** (→). (Ref: Shopfner CE, Hutch JA: The normal urethrogram. *Radiol Clin North Am* 1968; 6:165.)

FIG 13–78.—Elevation and elongation of the bladder due to accumulation of large amounts of fat in the pelvis. See also Figures 11–159 and 11–160 for related effects on the colon. (Ref: Fogg LB, Smyth JW: Pelvic lipomatosis: A condition simulating pelvic neoplasm. *Radiology* 1968; 90:558.)

FIG 13–80.—The trigone of the bladder. *Top left,* 6-year-old boy. *Top right,* 8-year-old boy. *Bottom right,* 29-year-old woman.

FIG 13–81.—The "female prostate," an indentation in the base of the bladder produced by asymmetry of the symphysis pubis. (Ref: Pope TL Jr, et al: Bladder base impressions in women: "Female prostate." *AJR* 1981; 136:1105.)

FIG 13–82.—The prostatic utricle in an 8-year-old boy, not to be mistaken for a diverticulum.

FIG 13–83.—The plicae colliculi, not to be mistaken for valves.

FIG 13–84.—Two examples of normal intermuscular incisurae of the posterior urethra. **A,** 19-year-old man. **B,** 11-year-old boy. (Ref: Shopfner CE, Hutch JA: The normal urethrogram. *Radiol Clin North Am* 1968; 6:165.)

FIG 13–85.—Another example of intermuscular incisurae of the posterior urethra in an 11-year-old boy. **A,** urethra distended by retrograde injection. **B,** during voiding. Note shadow of the verumontanum (←) and mucosal folds (⇷).

FIG 13–86.—**A,** voiding film. The external sphincter (→) and the insertion point of the suspensory ligament of the penis (↠) should not be mistaken for areas of organic narrowing. **B,** retrograde examination.

FIG 13–87.—Cowper's glands, not to be mistaken for false passages.

FIG 13–88.—Finger pressure producing an apparent stricture of the urethra. A similar defect can be produced by pressure by the lip of the collecting receptacle. (Ref: Lebowitz RL: Pseudostricture of the urethra: Urinal artefact on urethrography. *AJR* 1978; 130:570.)

FIG 13–89.—The "spinning top" urethra in a 6-year-old girl. This is believed to be a normal apparance seen in forceful voiding and is not the product of distal obstruction. (Ref: Whitaker J, Johnson GS: Correlation of urethral resistance and shape in girls. *Radiology* 1968; 91:757.) It has been stated that this configuration is the result of unstable contractions that are resisted by a voluntary increase in distal sphincter tension to prevent leakage of urine and that it does not represent a normal variant. (Ref: Saxton HM, et al: Spinning top urethra: Not a normal variant. *Radiology* 1988; 168:147).

FIG 13–90.—Phleboliths in the corpora cavernosa in a 40-year-old man, simulating urethral calculi.

FIG 13–91.—Intravaginal voiding. **A,** cystogram. **B,** vaginal residue.

FIG 13–92.—The arcuate uterus seen by hysterosalpingography. The impression in the fundus was misinterpreted as a myoma.

FIG 13–93.—Normal filling of the endocervical glands on hysterosalpingography.

Index